Frameworks of Choice

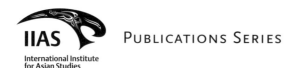

PUBLICATIONS SERIES

The *IIAS Publications Series* consists of Monographs and Edited Volumes. The Series publishes results of research projects conducted at the International Institute for Asian Studies. Furthermore, the aim of the Series is to promote interdisciplinary studies on Asia and comparative research on Asia and Europe.

The *International Institute for Asian Studies* (IIAS) is a postdoctoral research centre based in Leiden and Amsterdam, the Netherlands. Its objective is to encourage the interdisciplinary and comparative study of Asia and to promote national and international cooperation. The institute focuses on the humanities and social sciences and, where relevant, on their interaction with other sciences. It stimulates scholarship on Asia and is instrumental in forging research networks among Asia scholars worldwide.
IIAS acts as an international mediator, bringing various parties together, working as a clearinghouse of knowledge and information. This entails activities such as providing information services, hosting academic organisations dealing with Asia, constructing international networks, and setting up international cooperative projects and research programmes. In this way, IIAS functions as a window on Europe for non-European scholars and contributes to the cultural rapprochement between Asia and Europe.

For further information, please visit www.iias.nl.

Frameworks of Choice

Predictive & Genetic Testing in Asia

Edited by Margaret Sleeboom-Faulkner

AMSTERDAM UNIVERSITY PRESS

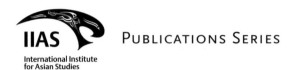

PUBLICATIONS SERIES

International Institute
for Asian Studies

EDITED VOLUMES 3

Cover illustration: Photograph by Margaret Sleeboom-Faulkner

Cover design: Maedium, Utrecht
Layout: The DocWorkers, Almere

ISBN   978 90 8964 165 6
e-ISBN 978 90 4851 117 4
NUR   870

© IIAS / Amsterdam University Press, Amsterdam 2010

Contents

Acronyms

ADR	Adverse drug reaction
AIIMS	All India Institute of Medical Sciences
ABI	Association of British Insurers
IFSA	Australian Investment and Financial Services Association
CP	Cerebral palsy
CDCP	Centre for Disease Control and Prevention
CH	Congenital hypothyroidism
CF	Cystic fibrosis
DM	Diabetes mellitus
DNA	Deoxyribonucleic acid
DS	Down's Syndrome
DMD	Duchenne muscular dystrophy
EQAS	External Quality Assurance Scheme
FDA	Food and Drug Administration
FOSHU	Food for Specified Healthcare Use
GAIC	Genetics and Insurance Committee
GINA	Genetic Information Non-disclosure Act
G6PH	Glucose-6-phosphate hydrogenase
HD	Huntington's Disease
HGP	Human Genome Project
ICMR	Indian Council for Medical Research
ISPAT	Indian Society for Prenatal Diagnosis and Therapy
IHA	International Huntington's Association
ILSI	International Life Sciences Institute
JIA	Japanese Insurance Association
MSS	Maternal Serum Sampling
MAM	Maharashtra Arogya Mandal
MD	Muscular dystrophy
NHGRI	National Human Genome Research Institute
OB	Obstetrician
PAASP	Parents Association for the Advancement of the Special Person
PRC	Peoples Republic of China
PKU	Phenyl ketonuria
PGT	Predictive genetic testing

PGD   Preimplantation genetic diagnosis
PND   Prenatal genetic diagnosis
SCA   Sickle Cell Anaemia
SNP   Single nucleotide polymorphism
SCA   Spino cerebellar ataxia
SMA   Spino muscular atrophy
SRGH   Sri Ganga Ram Hospital
TMS   Tandem Mass Spectrometry
USGAO   United States Government Accountability Office
WHO   World Health Organisation

Acknowledgements

This collection of case studies is the result of collaborative efforts of an international group of social scientists studying the impact of predictive and genetic testing on Asian society. They have exerted great efforts, both linguistically and in the area of theorising the socio-economic and cultural dimensions of predictive and genetic testing.

This volume would not have come about without the support and encouragement of the International Institute for Asian Studies in Leiden (IIAS), the Amsterdam School for Social Science Research (ASSR), the Genomics Initiative of the Netherlands Organisation for Scientific Research (NWO), and the Economic and Social Research Council (ESRC, RES-350-27-0002; RES-062-23-0215) in the UK. These organisations shouldered the expenses of the special symposium on 'Predictive Genetic Testing in Asia: social-science perspectives on the ramification of choice' at the 8th World Congress on Bioethics (8th WCB) in Beijing in August 2006, the double panel on *The quality of Offspring* held at the fifth edition of the International Convention of Asia Scholars in Kuala Lumpur in August 2007, and the conducted research and fieldwork in Asia out of which this volume has grown. Here I would also like to acknowledge the generosity of *The Journal of Bioethical Inquiry* (JBI), who gave permission for the rewriting and republication of two articles that appeared in a symposium of JBI in December 2007 as Chapters 2 and 3 in this volume. I also would like to express my gratitude to the book's English copy-editor Lee Bowers, the creator of the index, Cressida Jervis, and the reviewers and Barbara Prainsack, whose efforts and advice have been very much appreciated by all of the chapter contributors.

1 Frameworks of Choice

The Ramification of Predictive and Genetic Testing in Asia

Margaret Sleeboom-Faulkner

The rapid global expansion of predictive and genetic technologies is re-defining the meanings of health and healthcare, linking formulations of genetic identity to concepts of disease in terms of prevention, genetic therapy, personalised medicine and diet foods. This volume arose from the realisation that the significance of this global expansion in the field of predictive and genetic technologies in the context of Asian societies has not received the attention it deserves. The use of predictive and genetic testing (PGT) technologies in Asia is about the desire to understand current health statuses and situations, and the wish to have, or not to have, knowledge about future health. Health prospects are valued in various families, communities, societies and healthcare systems, and this leads to dilemmas for discussions attempting to generalise bioethical guidelines for the applications of PGTs. This is evident from a growing interest in the ethical questions that surround the new technologies. Indeed, accompanying the globalisation of advanced biomedical research, bioethical discussions on the interaction between biotechnology and the community have proliferated over the last four decades, also in Asia. Thus, in Japan, kindled by American discourse, interest in bioethical issues regarding euthanasia, patient-doctor relations and informed consent has grown rapidly since the 1980s (Morioka 2004; Kimura 1993). In China, a bioethics movement is beginning to flourish, and is expected to gain momentum, especially after the establishment of the Chinese Bioethics Association in October 2007. Additionally, bioethics discussions by overseas Chinese, Hong Kong, Singapore and Taiwan have stimulated the development of a body of what is regarded as typically Chinese/Asian thinking about bioethics, sometimes supported by other Asian nation-states such as Japan and South Korea (Qiu 2006; Döring 1999; Fan 1999). The same held true for Islamic schools of bioethics, which are sprouting in India, Malaysia, Singapore and Pakistan but receive a major incentive from universities in Europe and the US.[1] Social movements interested in bioethics flourish, especially in the wealthier parts of Asia, and in particular among intellectuals.[2]

The recognition of different cultural and religious values and the establishment of a new bioethics alone cannot lead to an adequate understanding of the issues involved in the application of newly developed biomedical technologies. This edited volume aims to introduce and provide examples of social science approaches applied to practices of predictive genetic testing in Asia. The book tries to make clear that without adequate insight into the unintended socio-economic consequences of government policies and regulation, and without the awareness of socio-political inequalities across national borders, even the most superior bioethical thinking and policies are of no avail to the lives of the genetically 'unfortunate' in any cultural context.

The development of new reproductive and genetic technologies (NRGTs) has made possible the predictive (including prenatal and genetic) testing for a range of monogenetic disorders, such as Down's syndrome, Duchenne muscular dystrophy (DMD), and Huntington's disease (HD). NRGTs in the future will also provide genetic information to large human groups for a variety of multiple-factor genetic disorders. This information, however, has an increasingly higher margin of uncertainty. Thus, susceptibility screening (e.g. for cancer, cardiovascular diseases, and neuropsychiatric diseases) will require analysis of multiple genes as well as environmental factors, such as lifestyle and living conditions. A high margin of uncertainty will yield bioethical dilemmas to potentially 'presymptomatic' groups of people, and may lead to anxieties and difficulties regarding the long-term decisions people make in their lives. Discussion of these dilemmas has especially become urgent with the recent use of 'comparative genomic microanalysis' in hospitals in the United States, using gene chips to detect subtle chromosomal variations for the diagnosis of over 150 genetic diseases in the foetus (Anonymous 2008).

Especially when no cures or therapies are available, when people do not have the financial means to pay for healthcare, or when the financial and social consequences of a positive test outcome are an overwhelming burden, even the decision to take a test may be a dramatic one. Whereas to some, a genetic test offers the possibility of a disease-free life or the assurance of knowing what will come, others regard taking a test as potentially annihilating life's meaning. In the case of a late-onset disorder such as HD, for which there is no cure, its announcement might render life meaningless (Konrad 2005). In the case of prenatal testing, diagnosis may lead to difficult decisions to be made about the abortion of the foetus. The circumstances and socio-economic backgrounds in which people decide to undergo a test and in which they make reproductive choices is referred to here as *frameworks of choice*. The ways in which people deal with such 'choices' can only be understood in the light of the experience people have with disease and their ways of coping. These are referred to here as the *ramifications of choice*.

The concept of the 'framework of choice' puts into perspective approaches that regard 'individual' or 'autonomous choice' as the basis of predictive and reproductive decision-making, and provides a complementary alternative. The 'framework of choice' proceeds from the idea that choices are always preconditioned by socio-economic circumstances, opportunities, and the understanding thereof, including education, belief, social networks, employment, and political freedom. According to a 'framework of choice' approach to PGT, then, choices are a product of circumstances and structural factors, which delimit and condition the choices individuals, families and communities make. Thus, classic approaches to bioethics focusing on 'individual choice' derive from comparatively narrow notions of choice. Although 'individual choice' here is not a concept criticised for its focus on the individual regarding decision-making, the cases in this collected volume do show the necessity of understanding the 'frameworks of choice' of individuals in order to understand their 'freedom of choice'. Furthermore, such 'frameworks of choice' also throw light on the conceptual frameworks, including historical and cultural narratives and political discourse, in which choices are formulated and bioethical notions are understood.

Varying cultural, economic and political conditions lead to different testing practices, different ramifications of choice, and therefore different ideas about bioethics. Asian countries harbour a great variety regarding population policies, family organisation, gender distinctions, views on the value of the embryo and life, medical health provision, and regulatory policies in the field of reproductive medicine. Furthermore, ramifications of bioethical choice in Asian societies, as in other societies, are couched in terms of cultural categories at the same time that they are conditioned by these categories. For instance, various cultural/religious norms may be used in encouraging or discouraging prospective parents to terminate pregnancy. Thus, depending on the environment and circumstances, questions that physicians and nurses ask could culturally condition a pregnant woman's choice: Don't you want the best for your child? Do you want your child to become a burden to society? Do you believe God would want you to respect the life you are carrying? To understand how cultural factors are related to choice, we need to gain insight into the meaning and implications of the use of cultural categories of 'abnormality'. If we hope to increase our understanding of reproductive diseases within the context of prenatal testing, we need to know how these cultural/religious categories relate to other 'hidden' social and personal motivations.

The next sections of this introduction are meant to provide a conceptual background to some of the technical terms used in this volume.

The first section defines various forms of genetic and predictive testing (PGT) and the second introduces the authors and their chapters. The concluding chapter of this volume contains an analysis of the main themes discussed in the volume.

Forms of genetic and predictive testing

This section on ethical and social considerations related to different forms of predictive and genetic testing (PGT) discusses terms used in the contributions on genetic and predictive testing, and aims to stimulate discussion on the economic and socio-cultural nature of the problems associated with PGT in Asian societies. I begin with 'standard' definitions of prenatal testing/screening, carrier/predictive testing and population/genetic screening. It should be pointed out, however, that such standard definitions proceed from an ideal-typical society in which healthcare is accessible, genetic counselling is provided and patients can make informed and voluntary decisions about having a test. However, as I go on to argue in the following sections, the definitions of which genetic abnormalities are worth screening for vary widely, and are decided in divergent manners by individuals, communities and nation-states (Mao & Wertz 1997; Mao 1998; Fujiki 2008; Unnithan 2006; Chee & Chan 1984).

Prenatal genetic diagnosis

Prenatal genetic diagnosis (PND) is a technique used to inform couples who are at increased risk of having a child with a genetic 'disorder' about the condition of a foetus or embryo. The diagnosis may help them decide whether to terminate the pregnancy or to prepare for the birth of a child with a disability. Risk factors might include advanced maternal age, a family history of a serious heritable medical condition, one or both parents being 'carriers' of mutation(s) in the same gene, abnormal test results such as ultrasound or first- and-second trimester screening tests, and a history of a previous child affected by a serious growth, developmental or health problem. *Antenatal or prenatal screening* provides prospective parents and healthcare professionals with information regarding the condition of the developing foetus. Prenatal screening includes a variety of procedures. Checking for a history of infertility, miscarriage, or a family history of genetic diseases might yield insight into current problems of infertility or risk of miscarriage; maternal serum screening tests may indicate possible genetic and/or structural defects in the baby; ultrasound scans of the foetus may detect structural abnormalities indicating possible genetic defects in the baby; and amniocentesis, to detect fetal abnormality, is an invasive procedure associated with risk of fetal damage (cf. Tsuge). PND can be carried out to identify specific genetic conditions, including Down's syndrome, thalassaemia and haemophilia.

Antenatal screening is a procedure intended to identify pregnancies in which the foetus has a serious malformation such as spina bifida, or a genetic condition such as Down's syndrome. In most societies with developed healthcare systems, maternal serum screening and ultrasound scanning are widely available. If a maternal serum screening indicates a certain probability of Down's syndrome, then amniocentesis may be offered as an option, even though this procedure has a risk of causing miscarriage. Depending on the country, however, a test may be relatively difficult to refuse (US; UK) or relatively difficult to obtain (Japan; the Netherlands) (Rapp 1999).

Carrier testing and predictive testing

Carrier testing is a method used to identify individuals who carry a genetic abnormality that does not affect the health of the person in question, but which increases the risk of producing offspring with a serious genetic disorder. Examples of such conditions include thalassaemia and muscular dystrophy (MD). Genetic counselling is normally recommended before and after the testing for such conditions, in order to prevent confusion over the difference between being an asymptomatic carrier – those who will not develop any signs of the disease – and being someone affected with it. In this regard, Peter Harper defined genetic counselling as 'the process by which patients or relatives at risk of a disorder that may be hereditary are advised of its consequences, the probability of developing and transmitting it and of the ways in which this may be prevented or ameliorated' (Harper 1988). Although genetic counselling aims to minimise adverse psychological reactions, it does not prevent carrier screening from creating opportunities for racial discrimination, as happened with sickle cell screening in the US in the 1970s (Lee 2003). Identified carriers can harbour lingering regrets and worries, while others may fail to recall the significance of their test result over time. More constructively, the information provided by carrier tests may be useful in family planning decisions, in the decision to have children, partner choice, and in preparing for the possibility of affected offspring (Prainsack & Siegal 2006; Brandt-Raouf 2006). Considering the serious impact of the outcome of carrier testing and the need for careful consideration of potential carriers and their families, the exploitation of this area of testing by commercial companies has been controversial. For this reason, there is a need to study the practices and motives of commercial carrier screening and the state health sector for offering tests (Sui & Sleeboom-Faulkner 2007).

Predictive testing identifies otherwise healthy individuals who have inherited a gene for a late-onset disease. A distinction can be made between presymptomatic testing and susceptibility testing. *Presymptomatic tests* identify healthy individuals who have inherited a defect in a specific gene for a late-onset disease, with an almost 100% risk of developing the disease. However, these tests usually cannot identify the severity and the time of onset of the disease. Examples of such diseases are Huntington's disease (HD) and cystic fibrosis, which are *monogenetic disorders* (single-gene disorders). *Susceptibility (or predisposition) tests* identify individuals who have inherited a genetic variant or variants, which may increase their risk of developing a *multifactorial disease*, due to the interaction of genes and the environment. Although very common, multifactorial diseases such as Alzheimer's disease, bowel cancer, breast cancer, heart disease, diabetes, hypertension and dementia are still little understood. Whilst technology can identify those at risk of disease, it is clearly problematic that there is no way of preventing it or improving treatment. There is, therefore, a 'therapeutic gap', which leaves those at increased risk for common diseases in a state of distress, denial and with inappropriate feelings of fatalism, and which might open up the possibility of discrimination (Simpson and Gupta).

Population genetic screening programmes

Genetic screening is defined by the WHO as 'tests offered to a population group to identify asymptomatic people at an increased risk from a particular adverse outcome' (WHO 1998). Genetic screening, then, is a diagnostic technique applied to a whole population, or to a distinct subgroup within a population, such as newborn infants or pregnant women. Genetic screening can be used to prevent a disease and/or minimize morbidity through early diagnosis and treatment. As screening tests are not definitive, a confirmatory diagnostic test is performed soon after a positive screening test result. This is important to prevent unnecessary anxiety and to enable measures for the prevention or treatment of the condition (Patra & Sleeboom-Faulkner 2008).

Although a simple idea in theory, the use of *population genetic screening programmes* is riddled with context-related bioethical problems. For example, is it ethical to offer such tests when there are no proven methods of treatment or prevention (Simpson, Gupta)? Where carried out without appropriate support in place, screening programmes may have risk implications for family members of the person screened (Patra & Sleeboom-Faulkner 2008). The process of giving information and obtaining consent should be tailored to the level of risk and benefit to the individual and the society. Some forms of prenatal and neonatal screening are provided routinely in countries with high standards of health-care provision and socio-cultural acceptance of their implementation (Tsuge, Kato). In the Asian Pacific area, neonatal screening programmes for important congenital diseases are well-established in some regions, but not so in others. Although the large geographical area and vast ethnic diversity contribute to variation in frequencies of congenital diseases in different regions, some diseases are commonly found in many regions. Examples are the thalassaemias, sickle cell anaemia (SCA), congenital hypothyroidism (CH) and glucose-6-phosphate dehydrogenase (G6PD) deficiency.

Examples of programmes used in some Asian countries include *antenatal screening* for Down's syndrome, and neonatal or newborn screening for G6PD deficiency to reduce the risk of neonatal jaundice and its complications, thalassaemia, sickle cell anaemia (SCA), phenylketonuria (PKU) and hearing defects, many of which are likely to be genetic in origin (Lam & Pang 1996). Potential advantages of presymptomatic screening include the ability to plan for the future, but these advantages may be offset against the distress of an early diagnosis. Yet, attitudes to detecting an inherited handicap appear to vary with the type of handicap. For instance, according to research conducted in Hong Kong, about 20 per cent of the general population felt that predictive screening was required for 'low intelligence', whereas about 70 to 90 per cent supported screening for cystic fibrosis and Down's syndrome (Lam & Pang 1996). Attitudes in families and among support groups also vary substantially, with some parents taking the line that 'family uncertainty about the future is reduced' and others taking the opposite view, that 'predictive screening should not be done just for the parents' peace of mind'. Similarly, widely diverging views on the influence of predictive testing on family life vary from 'high parental expectations of the child's behaviour are adjusted' to 'testing will destroy the innocence of childhood' and from 'doctors should be able to refuse tests in order to protect the child' to 'doctors should have no say in the matter' (Hjelm 1996).

In general, the bioethical problems associated with the application of PGTs are not exceptional compared to other forms of medical diagnosis. Usually, the introduction of predictive/genetic testing is meant to prevent harm and suffering, and to enable prospective parents and patients to make informed decisions. Yet, concerns remain that the introduction of a genetic test is not always based on evidence that the gene(s) examined is (are) associated with the disease in question. Furthermore, it is not always clear that the test itself has clinical validity and is useful to the people being tested (Sui & Sleeboom-Faulkner 2007; Wallace). The choice of a genetic test should be based on the individual's best interest *and* reflect his/her social values (Marteau & Johnston 1986; Henneman et al 2001). Apart from these relatively obvious issues and principles, the use of PGTs also has *unintended effects* that may be harmful to individuals and lead to discriminatory practices. For example, genetic information can lead to various forms of exclusion in marriage, school and employment (Sui & Sleeboom-Faulkner), in insurance companies' practices (Porter), in the inability to access healthcare (Simpson, Lee and Gupta), in the inability to act upon it, in the moral scruples to abort a foetus with a genetic abnormality (Tsuge, Kato and Simpson) or in the unacceptability of giving birth to a handicapped child in the eyes of the community (Simpson and Sui & Sleeboom-Faulkner) (Nie 2005; Scharping 2003).

The authors and the chapters

The chapters in this volume explore some of the frameworks in which reproductive choices and choices regarding PGTs are made in various Asian societies, that is, Mainland China, Japan, India and Sri Lanka, in addition to perspectives on frameworks of choice that vary globally. The authors of this volume are from a diverse disciplinary background, varying from sociology (Azumi Tsuge, Jyotsna Gupta), cultural anthropology (Bob Simpson, Sandra Soo-jin Lee, Margaret Sleeboom-Faulkner) and political science (Masae Kato) to biomedicine (Ishwar Verma, Renu Saxena), genetics and society (Susan Wallace), physical anthropology (Prasanna Patra), law (Gerard Porter, Suli Sui) and philosophy and Sinology (Ole Döring). However, all authors focus on predictive and genetic testing from the point of view of empirical study of socio-economic groups in society, rather than bioethical or philosophical ideals. All of the authors have experience in conducting fieldwork in Asia and have previously published in the fields of Asian studies, genomics or bioethics.

Crucial to an understanding of the ramifications of choice, we need insight into how motivations are related to the material/social circumstances in which people think about the possible outcomes of predictive genetic tests. How does the unfolding of a foretold disorder affect the lives, work and ambitions of individuals and families in Asian cultures? How does it affect family relations? How are genetic test results treated – with confidentiality, with secrecy, with openness, as warning? What sense do communities make of the genetic test results and what are the consequences for carriers? What choices do prospective parents have in the light of their perception of the anticipated outcome of a prediction? How and why do they couch their views in bioethical terms? This volume, then, aims to acquire comparative insights into the various ramifications of choice in a number of Asian countries from a social science point of view.

The various authors of this volume then respond to the following key questions:

- To what extent is choice regarding predictive genetic testing in Asia shaped by financial, legal, cultural, social and political factors?
- How do people experience predictive genetic testing in Asian countries in terms of choice? How do these involve views of the self, family, work, community, and future expectations?
- How are personal choices related to population policies, healthcare access and birth regulation?
- How do global developments in biotechnology and predictive testing influence Asian countries' health choices and national and ethnic identities?

South Asia

The chapters on South Asia pay attention to the 'therapeutic gap' and the financial and family circumstances of couples and individuals making use of PGTs. In Chapter 2, entitled 'Filling the Therapeutic Gap: Prenatal Diagnostics and Termination in Sri Lanka', Bob Simpson discusses problems linked to prenatal genetic testing in Sri Lanka, given that the possibilities for acting upon it may be limited. This so-called 'therapeutic gap' is discussed in the light of the economic, cultural and political factors linked to the decision to undergo testing, the availability and access to therapy and the ethical and cultural aspects of terminating a pregnancy. Based on surveys of doctors and medical students conducted over the period of 1986-2006, and interviews of parents of children with Down's syndrome held in 2002-3, this chapter situates questions of choice and decision-making around predictive and genetic testing in a society with severe restraints on abortion. These include Buddhist and Christian beliefs about the whys behind the occurrence and hows of the dealing with inherited syndromes, and financial and technological constraints limiting the possibilities for ameliorating the circumstance of the handicapped and their families.

In Chapter 3, 'Private and Public Eugenics: Predictive Genetic Testing and Individual Choice', Jyotsna Agnihotri Gupta clarifies the roles of the public and individuals in reproductive decision-making and predictive testing. Gupta puts into perspective the claim made by epidemiologists and geneticists that genetics has an increasing role to play in public health policies and programmes. Within this perspective, genetic testing and screening are instrumental in avoiding the birth of children with serious, costly or untreatable disorders. Introducing a distinction between concepts of private and public eugenics, Gupta refers to the practice of prenatal diagnosis as an aspect of private eugenics when the initiative to test comes from the pregnant woman herself. Public eu-

genics, by contrast, involves testing initiated by the state or medical profession through (more or less) obligatory testing programmes. In practice, however, the two co-occur. Thus, the management of thalassaemia
exemplifies how private eugenics tends to move into the sphere of public eugenics. Gupta views the recently launched newborn screening programme, however, as an example of public eugenics. Her exploration of
the thin line separating individual choice and overt or covert coercion,
and between private and public eugenics, shows that the use of genetic
testing technologies will have serious and far-reaching implications for
cultural perceptions of health and disease and women's experience of
pregnancy, besides creating new ethical dilemmas and new professional
and parental responsibilities.

Prasanna Kumar Patra and Margaret Sleeboom-Faulkner in Chapter
4, 'Population Genetic Screening for Sickle Cell Anaemia among the
Rural and Tribal Communities in India: the Limitation of Socio-ethical
Choice', discuss the effects of different forms of health interventions regarding sickle cell anaemia (SCA) in four different ethnographic sites.
Drawing on primary data collected through anthropological fieldwork
among scheduled tribe and caste communities, this chapter concerns
the difficulties around population genetic screening for SCA among tribal and rural communities in India. SCA is a genetically inherited disorder especially prevalent among Indian tribal and caste communities.
Population genetic screening among marginalised rural and tribal communities brings about social and ethical dilemmas over healthcare policy choices. Thus, stigmatisation has come about as a result of the discriminatory practices following the leaking and sometimes open announcement of test results. This chapter, then, problematises the lack
of attention to ethical principles in publicly mandated genetic screening
programmes. The authors contend that screening programmes for SCA
in rural and tribal areas in India are based on haphazard planning, leading to widespread discrimination and stigmatisation. Often, local communities have only little say in the question of whether the village is to
undergo a genetic test or screening. It is especially such ill-planned interventions, in which the local population has little say, which are
shown to generate new forms of inequality.

The authors of Chapter 5, Ishwar C. Verma and Renu Saxena, from
Sir Ganga Ram Hospital in New Delhi, have provided genetic counselling to several thousand families with diverse genetic disorders, including adult-onset genetic disorders. This experience has given them unique insight into the ethical and social issues related to predictive testing in a multiethnic and multicultural country such as India. In
'Predictive Genetic Testing – a Perspective from India', the authors discuss several ethical issues occurring in predictive testing for monogenetic disorders with adult onset, but which do not have any specific

treatment at present. Counsellors and physicians need to be extremely careful when offering predictive genetic tests in India, due to widely differing educational levels, and cultural and social beliefs. In a situation in which there are no formal guidelines for predictive testing, the authors decided to evaluate attitudes towards the testing in relation to social and religious values. In a survey on attitudes of patients/family members who had tested positive for HD, the authors explored questions related to family history, the decision to undergo a test, family support and information sharing, and effects of the tests on daily life and future planning. Their analysis of the survey examines the double-edged sword of genetic testing for various disorders in an Indian context: the consequences of a positive outcome, a negative one and not knowing are discussed in various cultural and medical scenarios in which family, socio-economic status and the availability of therapies play a major role.

Japan

In Chapter 6 on 'Genetic Testing: The Belief in Autonomous Decision-making among Japanese Women', Azumi Tsuge analyses the frameworks of choice from which Japanese women proceed in making reproductive decisions after ultrasound examination in Japan. In Japan, ultrasound examination during pregnancy is conducted frequently, as compared to the US. Yet the frequency of maternal serum screening tests and/or amniocentesis is relatively low. This phenomenon is due to historical and current socio-cultural influences, which are the subject of exploration in this chapter. Tsuge sets out by analysing the reasons for Japanese women to undergo prenatal testing, on the basis of a large-scale survey and interviews with doctors and women in the Tokyo areas in 2003-4, as a part of the project 'Women's Experiences of Pregnancies and Prenatal Tests'. Explaining the outcome of this survey, Tsuge refers to the limitations of the Eugenic Protection Law on the right of disabled people to have children. Partly as a response to this, Japan also has an ongoing history of the disabled rights movement severely criticising prenatal testing, such as amniocentesis, as a form of eugenics. Nevertheless, as medical technologies have developed rapidly over the last three decades, the number of women who undergo prenatal tests is increasing greatly. Despite the availability of technological know-how, both women and gynaecologists tend to avoid disclosure of the procedures so as to deflect criticism of discrimination against disabled people. This situation, Tsuge argues, differs fundamentally from considerations that influence reproductive decision-making in other countries, such as the US.

In Chapter 7, 'Cultural Notions of Disability and Prenatal Testing in Japan', Masae Kato discusses the views of ordinary citizens on disabilities and explores their relevance to the decision of individuals regarding prenatal testing. Prenatal testing here includes maternal serum sampling and amniocentesis. The majority of visitors to obstetricians are 'ordinary citizens', are politically unaffiliated, without professional medical knowledge, or have never previously been confronted with issues of disability. With scant medical knowledge, they find themselves face to face with obstetricians. The chapter examines six cases of pregnancy. Although unaware of belonging to a high-risk group, all expressed anxieties about the health of the foetuses during pregnancy. Three of the women underwent prenatal testing and three of them did not. Kato, in this chapter, analyses the motivations of individuals to undergo prenatal tests, taking into consideration their views on disabilities. Explanations regarding the cultural aspects of disability in Japan are made in the light of previous empirical studies on prenatal testing, as well as other sociological, anthropological and folklore studies regarding health, abnormality, reproduction and the family. It appears that the practice of ancestor worship (*senzo sūhai*) and blood ties are particularly helpful in explaining cultural perspectives on disability, and are important factors in explaining attitudes to predictive testing. The analysis demonstrates a prevailing naïveté among couples about the risks of pregnancy in Japan. Kato also highlights cases in which individuals are stigmatised in society due to ignorance about the aetiology of disability. She argues that these Japanese notions of ancestor worship, blood ties and disability are important to communication about pregnancy, not only at home, but in the hospital as well.

In Chapter 8, entitled 'Is Japan Ready for Genetic Testing? Balancing Public and Private Interests in the Context of Insurance', Gerard Porter sheds light on discussions and problems around genetic testing in relation to insurance companies, focusing on groundbreaking court cases which are expected to set a precedent for the role of genetic testing in relation to healthcare in Japanese society. In contrast to the position within most advanced industrial states, Japan has yet to implement laws and guidelines to regulate the use of genetic information by insurance companies. With the first example of civil litigation in the area of genetics and insurance having already reached the Japanese courts, this chapter examines whether the existing Japanese legal framework is sophisticated enough to manage the more widespread use of the results of genetic tests by insurers in the coming years. Confusion and conflicts of interest exist about the issue of who should take responsibility for the expenses related to genetic diseases and life insurance, when symptoms appear before the contract with the insurance company commenced, but whose genetic nature was not known beforehand. Porter discusses the implications for the provision of healthcare and the pressures on individuals to undergo predictive genetic tests.

China

In Chapter 9, 'Genetic Testing on DMD and Vulnerability of DMD Family in China – Case Studies of DMD families in Chinese Contexts', Suli Sui and Margaret Sleeboom-Faulkner describe the current practices of genetic testing on Duchenne muscular dystrophy (DMD) and the difficulties faced by DMD families in a Chinese context, drawing on interviews with geneticists, doctors working in the clinic as genetic counsellors and the families of DMD patients. Using four case studies, the chapter focuses on the implications of genetic counselling and testing on DMD for reproductive decision-making and life planning in conjunction with the influence of Chinese family planning policies, economic conditions, distribution of health resources, the healthcare system and Chinese culture. This constellation of factors, playing a major role in generating anxiety regarding carrier testing and disability, requires a rethink of socio-political and economic issues related to social stigma, healthcare access, education and social support and help for children with DMD and their families. The chapter shows how the application of genetic technology to a certain extent improves the situation of DMD families in China, but at the same time makes the DMD patients and their families vulnerable to discrimination, social isolation and financial difficulties.

In Chapter 10, on 'Ramifications of Choice: Ethical, Cultural and Social Dimensions of Sex Selection in China', Ole Döring discusses sex selection in China, and debates on sex selection from the perspective of free choice. This approach, one often defended by utilitarian views on sex selection, Döring regards as methodologically inadequate as well as ethically barren. Building on empirical studies about the phenomenon of 'missing girls' and gender discrimination, the chapter analyses relevant cultural and ethical circumstances and discusses recent governance measures regarding sex selection and their consequences for reproductive choices in China. The chapter's main argument is that, in contemporary China, it would be inappropriate to assess the issues of sex selection in terms of 'freedom of choice' or as the 'individual's right to independent procreative decision-making'. Any attempt to declare the de facto practice in China at face value as an expression of individual, social or cultural self-determination is flawed, and would be unsympathetic to the affected population.

Asia and the global arena

In Chapter 11, 'Genetic Testing and Diet-related Disease in Asia: Preventing Diseases or Misleading Marketing?', Helen Wallace examines the influence of diet in commercial attempts to push lucrative remedies for diet-related genetic diseases. Predictive genetic testing is expanding to include tests for genetic susceptibility to common diseases such as heart disease and type 2 diabetes. One proposed application of these tests is in 'personalised nutrition', combining genetic tests with dietary advice, including advice to take dietary supplements or to eat functional foods. Personalised nutrition is being advocated as a solution to the global epidemic of diet-related diseases, an epidemic expected to have particularly serious health consequences in Asia. So far it is questionable whether personalised nutrition will reduce the incidence of these diseases. The two main concerns are that, firstly, genetic tests and functional foods are targeted at the relatively wealthy and do nothing to help lower socio-economic groups or people in poorer countries; and, secondly, biology is too complex, making individual risks inevitably uncertain and hard to predict, and limiting the usefulness of targeting lifestyle advice at 'high-risk' individuals. Wallace discusses two important issues arising within the context of the future market for predictive genetic testing in Asia: whether personalised nutrition, nutritional genetics and genomics are good priorities for health research, and whether health claims for genetic tests and associated food products are likely to be adequately regulated.

In Chapter 12 on 'Pharmacogenomic Medicine in Asia and the Geneticisation of National Identity', Sandra Soo-Jin Lee shows how several nations, including the US and the UK, have recently focused on persistent health disparities among their own racially and ethnically identified populations, but have paid little attention to the potential impact of genomic technologies on global health disparities. This chapter explores the ethical and social implications of pharmacogenomic developments, and the emerging framework of genomic-driven Asian identities, in the framework of an increasingly racialised global context. It explores the question of how the availability of DNA samples from Asia impacts the scientific research and discovery of population-specific markers of drug response. The chapter further examines the current infrastructure for pharmacogenomic development in Asia and how it will affect current global disparities in healthcare. In grappling with these questions, Lee discusses current trends, impediments and possibilities in pharmacogenomics and the development of therapeutic drugs intended to be more efficacious and less toxic in Asian individuals. In short, Lee discusses the institutional forces exacerbating the fault lines of population-based therapeutics, and their impact on the ability of individuals to reap the promised benefits of genomic medicine.

The concluding chapter discusses the main themes of this volume in relation to frameworks of choice. The chapter first discusses the extent to which 'free' will or 'free' choice can be said to determine the termination of pregnancy, and relates 'free' will to socio-economic and cultural considerations and conditions. These in turn form the basis of the second section, a discussion of the financial, cultural and religious spaces opened up by therapeutic gaps. The third theme concerns the role of the state as a variable factor, co-determining the way PGTs develop in relation to other social, financial and cultural factors. The fourth theme of culture is discussed in relation to discrimination and the stigma attached to the handicapped and their families. In this socio-cultural field, it becomes clear how in various countries the role of the state, healthcare provision and local power relationships are crucial to the way in which PGTs develop. Also, the role of the market, the fifth theme of the chapter, plays fundamentally different roles in shaping the benefits and risks of the multiple ways in which PGTs develop in local contexts. The role of the pharmaceutical industry in genomic research and in sampling and testing activities is discussed in the last section.

Notes

1   E.g. Sachedina A. Available: http://people.virginia.edu/~aas/home.htm
2   See Eubios. Available: www.eubios.info/

2   A 'Therapeutic Gap'

Anthropological Perspectives on Prenatal Diagnostics and Termination in Sri Lanka

Bob Simpson

Introduction

Rapid advances in biotechnology and an ever more sophisticated capacity to 'read' genes and chromosomes are providing startling insights into the human condition. Conditions and dispositions that might hitherto have been understood in terms of unassailable fate, chance and destiny might now be explained using the gene as the determining agent par excellence. Crucial in this respect is the proliferation of predictive genetic testing, an expanding ensemble of techniques in which blood or tissue is used to identify genetic diseases (see Sleeboom-Faulkner this volume, Chapter 1). The power of this kind of testing, however, is not just that it offers the possibility of knowing why things are as they are in the present but, more crucially, how they might unfold across lifetimes and, indeed, across generations. Testing genes and chromosomes is thus a future-oriented act; it invites speculation, and estimation of what might come to pass.

Whilst the means currently becoming available to glimpse the future might be novel, the motivation to do so is anything but. The ubiquitous arts of divination, foretelling, augury and prediction have long been the hallmark of a specifically human creative endeavour, in which attempts are made to conceive of a person's future from signs available in the present. Entrails, piles of sticks, playing cards, the movement of the planets, the lines on one's hand – the ways in which humans have sought to get some purchase on destiny would make for a very long list. This knowledge has a powerful motive force as it passes from expert exponents of the 'test' and into the life-worlds of ordinary people in the form of diagnosis and prognosis (see for example Latimer 2007). Such knowledge cannot just be for its own sake but, because it is always to some degree partial and contingent, invites interpretation, elaboration and supplementary action believed to maximise well-being and good fortune and mitigate suffering and misfortune. Here we enter the existentially compelling world of human circumstance, and the complex actions and beliefs that are brought into play in the quest for order and meaning in the face of actual or potential suffering. Techniques such as prenatal genetic diagnosis (PND) and, more recently, preimplantation genetic diagnosis (PGD), although highly advanced technological interventions, thus represent a point of crossover into the worlds of mundane decision-making, which constitute people's day-to-day lives. At this point of encounter, we also enter the domain, often obscured by the abstractions to which bioethical discourse is prone, in which the social sciences have a significant part to play. Anthropological approaches, and particularly the holism which ethnography invites, provide new dimensions to bioethical inquiry. Such approaches do not necessarily provide clear answers but offer the possibility of understanding the consequences that technologies have in circumstances that are 'multipartite, relational and complex' (Franklin & Roberts 2006: 9).

Paying attention to the ways in which the encounter with the technologies of prenatal testing takes place in different socio-cultural settings provides important insights into the way these technologies are socialised, politicised and rendered culturally appropriate. In short, it highlights the ways in which society and culture might be made visible in our attempts to understand what reproductive ethics might encompass in different settings. The scientific specificity of knowledge produced by means of a biomedical procedure with the label 'test' comes at the point where actual pasts and possible futures meet, not just for individuals but also for wider networks of kin and community. Thus, genetic testing is not separate from but already entwined with pre-existing ideas of fate and destiny. Between technological possibility and normative constraint, people must construct an everyday ethics to enable them to proceed in ways that are coherent and meaningful. The 'test' has social, cultural and political dimensions, and we need to look much wider than the 'narrowing scope of the clinical gaze' (Good 1994: 180) if we are to make sense of the global engagement with the biosciences in general and genetic testing in particular (Rapp 1999; Franklin & Roberts 2006).

In this essay, I consider the nature of this engagement in the context of contemporary Sri Lanka. At the present time in Sri Lanka, prenatal diagnostic testing provides a highly sought-after degree of foresight. Reproduction, and moreover, reproduction of healthy children, is a much valued achievement which is willed with deep passion by couples and their extended families. However, the production of information about the state of the embryo or the foetus yields knowledge that can prove deeply problematic, given that the possibilities for acting upon it may be limited. In other contexts this problematic has been referred to as the 'therapeutic gap': the discrepancy that exists between diagnosis and the options available for therapeutic intervention (Holtzman & Shapiro 1998; Nordgren 2001: 179; Andrews 2001: 5). In the context of genetic testing, this discrepancy is not small, as the idea of a 'gap' might suggest, but a yawning chasm between the ever-growing repertoire of tests for genetic diseases and conditions on the one hand, and the narrow range of options available to mitigate, combat or eliminate these on the other. As an object of study, the 'therapeutic gap' has multiple dimensions – ethical, social, cultural and economic – and the question of whether under any one set of circumstances the gap is widened or narrowed depends on the pulling and pushing of all these factors. Some attempts to bridge the genetic 'therapeutic gap' are non-controversial, and involve the provision of services and support to help parents manage the arrival of a child with a genetic condition. As parents are also eager to learn what the birth of one child might mean for the birth of the next, guidance over future reproductive decisions is also likely to be provided. Other actions, however, are more controversial; in particular, the use of termination as a 'therapeutic' option. Strangely, reference to termination is often absent from discussions of prenatal genetic testing and is usually passed off euphemistically as an aspect of reproductive choice. In this essay, I focus on the relationship between genetic testing and termination, exploring the interface between the 'public' and 'private' parameters of reproductive choice, that is, the legal and cultural factors defining reproductive choice in the context of contemporary Sri Lanka.

The particular elements that I am interested to explore in the Sri Lankan context are threefold:

1. There is a strong prohibition on taking life and hence on termination of pregnancy.
2. There is widespread support among professionals and public alike for a limited liberalisation of the laws relating to termination, particularly where serious genetic disorders are identified.
3. There is a popular preoccupation with a variety of systems and signs that are commonly used to read present and future states of health and well-being.

These three elements are often found blended together in people's thinking about genetic testing. Here I hope to highlight some of the particularities emerging from this process and the distinctive version of the resulting 'therapeutic gap'. The first perspective I consider is that of doctors and medical students, surveyed at various points between 1986 and 2006 about their views on reproductive testing. The second is that of parents of children with Down's syndrome whom I encountered during research carried out into new reproductive and genetic technologies in 2002-03. First, however, a little by way of contextualisation is necessary.

The context

In Sri Lanka, as elsewhere in the developing world, there is a drive to engage with technologies to enable testing and screening for genetic disorders to occur. This drive comes from at least two sources.

First, it is propelled by a growing awareness of what has been characterised as an 'epidemiological' or 'demographic' transition (WHO 2002). The transition comes about as improved nutrition and control of infectious diseases in the developing world leads to falling childhood mortality rates. The result, it is argued, is the emerging visibility of a new global health problem, in the form of increasing numbers presenting with genetic disorders such as thalassaemia and other haemoglobinopathies (Weatherall & Clegg 2001). This observation has led to strong arguments that a 'genomic divide' is emerging, and that active strategies need to be in place if this is to be avoided (Singer & Daar 2001; WHO 2002). In Sri Lanka, for example, work on the incidence of thalassaemia has identified significant resource implications arising from long-term transfusion-dependent individuals, and an identified need to develop screening and counselling services (De Silva, Jayasekera & Rubasinghe 1997; De Silva, Fisher, Premwardhena et al 2000).

Second, Sri Lanka's engagement with cytogenetic and DNA technologies is driven by market forces. Put simply, there is a growing demand for highly specialised diagnostic services delivered via the private sector to those who can afford them. Currently, this demand is being catered to by a mixture of local private-sector initiatives as well as by an influx of foreign-backed clinics and hospitals opening up on Sri Lankan soil, offering tests for conditions such as beta thalassaemia, cystic fibrosis, Duchenne muscular dystrophy, haemophilia A and B, Fragile X syndrome, Down's syndrome and haemochromotosis. It is interesting in this regard to note that there has been a growing anxiety in Sri Lanka regarding the spread of medical diagnostic laboratories offering a wide range of tests and scans (Perera 2006). The concern is that large numbers of these laboratories cater not just to those who are ill, but prey upon those who are concerned about what might be wrong with them, a constituency familiar from other contexts as the 'anxious well'. It is not inconceivable that the penchant for testing will extend to the new range of prenatal diagnostics. The increased frequency of genetic testing has also given rise to concerns about the accuracy and appropriateness of testing in some settings (Dissanayake & Jayasekera 2008).

Both of these drivers – global public health concerns and market opportunities – are underpinned by Sri Lanka's increasing participation in the global commerce in scientific knowledge and technology. More specifically, the spectacular progress of close neighbours such as India, China and Korea in the field of biotechnology means that this commerce is no longer primarily Euro-American in its origins (Sleeboom-Faulkner 2004a). The engagement with these technologies brings with it a wide range of ethical and legal challenges. Over the last decade there has been a gradual mobilisation of committees, advisory groups and research concerned with the implications of genetic testing and manipulation (Simpson 2001; NASTEC 2003).

Although the technologies and expertise necessary to engage with testing for a wide repertoire of genetic conditions are subject to deliberation and debate, the wholehearted embrace of these powerful diagnostic tools in practice appears to be a long way off. As previously with amniocentesis and chorionic villus sampling, the new generation of genetic tests arouses ethical sensitivities, which make their introduction extremely problematic. In reproductive genetic testing, as it occurs in the West, there is an implicit link, widely taken for granted, between the results of genetic testing and the ability to act on those results by way of terminating a pregnancy. The new genetic technologies push the diagnosis of abnormality earlier and earlier, and with this comes a further assumption that moral qualms about termination will recede the earlier abnormalities can be detected (Lippman 1991). In many Western countries, where genetic abnormality and termination are concerned, the 'therapeutic gap' is not large and appears to be narrowed at every turn (for example, see Liu, Joseph, Kramer et al 2002).[1] In Sri Lanka, however, termination of pregnancy is to all intents and purposes illegal. Section 303 of the Penal Code of Sri Lanka states that termination of pregnancy is available only where a mother's health is directly threatened and three physicians are prepared to sign a form to this effect. Consequently, the linkage between testing and termination is simply not there in any official sense. The 'therapeutic gap' is effectively unbridgeable and there are powerful forces and interests keen to ensure that it remains so.

Preventing any potential linkage between testing and termination are deeply held religious convictions about the sanctity of life, and particularly those held by the Buddhist *sangha* and the Catholic Church. The orthodox position held by Theravada Buddhists in Sri Lanka is that consciousness does not develop over the course of gestation, but arrives fully formed at the point of conception when a force or energy (*viññāna*) from a previous incarnation arrives in the newly formed embryo. Prior to this event there is inanimate matter for which there is little by way of ethical concern, hence a rather liberal attitude towards barrier contraception, IVF and even reproductive cloning. However, following conception and implantation in the womb, life is present in the form of a being with a desire to live and to be reborn again; the consequences of failing to protect this life are serious, both in this life and beyond (Keown 1995; Harvey 2000). As one doctor interviewed put it: 'It doesn't matter how life originates as long as it is preserved once it has originated.' In other words, arguments about earlier abortion being less sinful don't hold for many orthodox Buddhists, who believe consciousness to be fully formed at the very earliest stages of human development. Although Christian notions of embryogenesis do not have anything akin to the arrival of the *viññāna*, the idea that the point of conception is the instant of ensoulment does result in significant parallels being drawn. This is particularly the case within Catholic doctrines. Such parallels go some way to explaining why, when over many other matters there is friction, Buddhist and Catholic clergy are strongly aligned in their opposition to termination of pregnancy, however close to conception it might happen to fall.

Yet, in other respects, the 'therapeutic gap' is disturbingly absent. Although termination in most circumstances remains strictly illegal, in practice things are quite different. Albeit clandestinely, abortion is widely available and, if estimates are correct, appears to take place with alarming frequency. Unofficial estimates put the number of terminations in the region of 700-1000 per day (De Soysa 2000). The majority of these terminations appear to be sought by older married women for whom contraception has failed (Deok, Jinhyun & De Silva 2002). Amongst these women there is a high rate of death (estimated between 10 and 30 per cent of all maternal deaths) due to septic abortion (Gunasekere & Wijesinha 2001). However, with the emergence of private clinics and hospitals, it is likely that women with the means to pay will, in fact, have relatively easy access to safe abortion, usually euphemistically described as 'menstrual regulation'. In short, with the law on termination as it stands, there is a major disjunction between what policy dictates and how citizens act. Attempts by women's groups and some branches of the medical profession to modify the Penal Code so that termination of pregnancy might be available in cases of rape, to unmarried mothers, in cases of incest or where there are fetal abnormalities have, to date, proved unsuccessful.

The medical profession in particular finds itself caught up in this disjunction. Colleagues in Sri Lanka have carried out survey work over a period of twenty years regarding the attitudes of doctors and medical students to prenatal diagnostic testing and termination. In 1986, a series of surveys were conducted to ascertain the views of doctors (n=302) and medical students (n=173) regarding amniocentesis, counselling and termination of pregnancy (Jayasekara 1986; Jayasekara, Kristl & Wertelecki 1988; Jayasekara 1989). As part of research into the reception of the new reproductive and genetic technologies in Sri Lanka, performed between 2000 and 2004, Simpson, working in collaboration with Jayasekera and Dissanayake of the University of Colombo Human Genetics Unit, replicated aspects of the earlier survey and added a series of new questions dealing with more recent developments relating to genetic technologies and the manipulation of gametes and embryos (Dissanayake, Simpson & Jayasekara 2002; Simpson, Dissanayake, Wickremasinghe & Jayasekera 2003; Simpson, Dissanayake & Jayasekera 2005). Again, doctors (n=278) and medical students (n=1256) were surveyed. The results of these surveys are presented in Table 2.1 in the form of simple descriptive statistics (Simpson et al 2005: Table 1). A more rigorous statistical analysis is available elsewhere (Simpson et al 2005). Each of these surveys reveals a significant tension between what doctors and medical students think should be allowed to happen and what is permitted to happen by law. Among doctors, the proportion in favour of

Table 2.1 *Attitudes towards prenatal diagnosis and therapeutic abortion in the 2002 survey*

	Percentage positive response	
	Doctors	Students
Amniocentesis significantly affects the usefulness of genetic counselling	73% (203) (94)*	80% (1008) (75)*
Amniocentesis is a good idea if a genetic disorder such as Down's syndrome has already appeared in the family	87% (242) (98)	87% (1093) (89)
Amniocentesis should be offered to all pregnant women over the age of 35 years if there is legal provision for therapeutic abortion	71% (198) (78)	78% (976) (72)
Amniocentesis should be offered to satisfy prenatal curiosity about the sex of the foetus	11% (30) (30)	27% (338) (32)
If by amniocentesis a gross genetic defect was detected an abortion might be appropriate	93% (259) (89)	81% (1013) (69)
Using preimplantation genetic diagnosis (PGD) is an acceptable way to screen for genetic disorders**	65% (181) –	70% (878) –
If yes, to previous question: If abnormalities are identified through PGD it is acceptable to discard the embryos**	84% (232) –	80% (1000) –
There should be provision made in the law to carry out a therapeutic abortion when a genetic defect is detected antenatally	87% (239) (96)	80% (1009) (88)
It will be a great achievement when genetic engineering of the human genome enables us to eliminate serious genetic defects	90% (249) –	90% (1132) –

* Figures in italics are the percentages reported for doctors and students in the 1986 survey.
** NB: these questions were not asked in the 1986 survey.

termination of pregnancy in circumstances where there is a gross genetic defect was broadly similar in the surveys carried out in 1986 and 2002 (Simpson et al 2005: Table 1). Of the doctors surveyed in 2002, 93 per cent (n=259) supported termination of pregnancy in such cases, compared with 89 per cent in the earlier survey (cf. De Silva et al 1997). Students appeared to support termination of pregnancy less than doctors, but comparison between the two samples indicates a much higher level of acceptance across the two surveys (81 per cent in the present sample as opposed to 69 per cent).

Consideration of preimplanatation genetic diagnosis (PGD) in relation to screening and possible termination of pregnancy in the 2002 survey revealed that, among doctors and students, approximately one-third were either against or undecided on the use of PGD for screening. It should be noted that questions about PGD were not asked in the 1986 survey, as a result of which data are missing from Table 2.1 (Simpson et al 2005: Table 1). The proportions in favour were 65 per cent of doctors and 70 per cent of students.

On the question of changing the law to allow termination in cases where there are genetic defects, 87 per cent of doctors and 80 per cent of students were in favour in the 2002 survey. These figures are of similar order to responses given in the 1986 survey (96 and 88 per cent, respectively). Written comments, which accompanied the various surveys suggest that, among doctors and students, there was a solid core of respondents drawn from each of the religious communities who were strongly opposed to allowing termination in these circumstances.

Compared with the 1984 survey, doctors' responses to the three questions regarding the use of amniocentesis would appear to be rather less positive than in the 2002 survey. In the 1986 survey, 94 per cent of doctors felt that amniocentesis significantly affected the potential usefulness of genetic counselling, whereas in the later survey only 73 per cent answered positively. Likewise, in relation to its use where there are already genetic disorders or the mother is older than 35, the proportions were lower (98 as compared to 87 per cent and 78 as compared to 71 per cent, respectively).

Several reasons might be put forward for the changing levels of enthusiasm regarding amniocentesis. It might be that concerns over the dangers accompanying such an invasive method might have increased over time and as more evidence about risks has become available. The decline in enthusiasm might thus be symptomatic of a growing conservatism in the use of certain interventions. Conversely, it may be that those interventions have simply been overtaken. Throughout the period in question, new techniques for detecting chromosomal abnormalities have appeared, such as chorionic villus sampling, new blood tests (for example, sampling alpha fetoprotein, oestriol and human chorionic gonadotrophin) and the measurement of nuchal fold using high-resolution ultrasound scanning. However, discussions with doctors regarding testing for Down's syndrome suggested another reason. For many, there was simply no point in engaging in testing which produced information that cannot then be acted upon. For them, there was not so much a 'therapeutic gap' as an enormous void. Indeed, it was considered by some to be deeply unethical to test under these circumstances. As one doctor put it in a written comment, 'No point doing amniocentesis when therapeutic abortion is not legalised.'

From the surveys carried out it is clear that, for some considerable time, the majority of doctors and students would like to have seen a more liberal relationship between testing and termination. However, the majority appear to be at odds with the minority of their colleagues, who oppose these changes on moral grounds but who are supported by the wider legal framework. Yet, as we have seen, the absence of termination as a legitimate option where serious genetic conditions are identified prenatally has played a significant part in preventing the uptake of prenatal testing in Sri Lanka and in turn limited the scope for genetic counselling despite an overwhelming recognition of its usefulness (De Silva et al 1997). As a consequence, it is possible that, as the next generation of genetic testing and screening becomes more easily available (e.g. in relation to thalassaemia or the dystrophies, such as Duchenne's disease), there will be a similarly partial and problematic engagement with testing and counselling in the public sector. To engage with the diagnostic and predictive powers of the new technologies would seem for many doctors to be a duty (to parents) and an obligation (to society) but, as long as it remains uncoupled from the possibility of reproductive choice, then there is little point in lobbying for resources to introduce testing and screening on any significant scale in the public sector, or to introduce the counselling necessary to assist parents in making informed choices. However, influential religious conservatism is not the only backdrop against which this dilemma is being played out. Marketisation of medical services and a concomitant growth of consumerist attitudes towards health have created expectations of greater freedom of choice, and not least when it comes to questions of reproduction. In the next section, I turn to a consideration of how these public and highly contentious dilemmas play out in the lives of those faced with significant reproductive dilemmas.

Down's syndrome: reading the signs

In November 2002, I attended a meeting of the Parents' Association for the Advancement of the Special Person (PAASP), a Sri Lankan support/pressure group for families in which there was a child with Down's syndrome.[2] At that time, the organisation was ground-breaking in that it was the first to mobilise the interests of such a community and had, as a result, attracted a great deal of interest from parents across the island. The organisation was in many regards a nascent expression of a growing disability rights movement that has begun to take shape in Sri Lanka in recent years. PAASP was active in lobbying for service provision and the mainstreaming of children with Down's syndrome in the education system; raising awareness and countering ignorance and prejudice through various publicity campaigns; and organising social events at which the parents of children with Down's syndrome could come together. Previously, parents of a child with Down's syndrome, or children with any other learning disability for that matter, have had little by way of information, emotional and practical support or a sense of a wider community of people with similar experiences. The sad reality is that these children are mostly treated as non-persons in Sri Lankan society [the use of the term 'special person' in the organisation's title is not without significance]. Parents typically experience isolation, stigma and significant hardship. It is not uncommon for people to stare or to pass comment when such children are encountered. Often, younger women will avoid physical or even visual contact for fear that such an inauspicious encounter will have a teratogenic effect upon their unborn children. Some parents talked of children being taunted or goaded and referred to by derogatory terms such as 'mongol' or 'China baby' (*mongol kiyanava* or *cheena babek*). For those who are Buddhists, there is usually the added burden of feeling that, in ways that they could never possibly know, parents themselves have contributed to their misfortune (*avasenava*) with the physical appearance of the child seen as public and incontrovertible evidence of a sin committed in a previous life (*pera kerapu pav* or *karumayak*). Whereas Christian parents of children with Down's syndrome with whom I have spoken have tended to see their circumstance as a special challenge or test from God, Buddhists, on the contrary, are more passive in their adversity, accepting the child as the working through of an all-embracing law of *karma* (Simpson 2007). For some parents, the consequences of their actions were thought to happen in a quite direct fashion, as in the case of the woman who linked in her mind the birth of her own child with the two abortions she had had before marriage. For others, *karma* was thought of in a far more nebulous fashion; it was simply enough to acknowledge that in some previous rebirth, parents and children had all done things, unspecified, that had moral consequences in this one.

At the PAASP meeting I attended, about a dozen active and enthusiastic parents had come together, as they did regularly, to exchange information and to organise their campaigns for improved services. The meeting began with one of the parents reporting that he had seen on the Internet a newly developed blood test that could detect trisomy-21 at an early stage. He emphasised that the test was simple and non-invasive. The discussion quickly turned to the question of testing and an issue that, collectively and individually, every parent in the room had clearly revisited time and again – would they have tested and what would they have done with the results? Knowing that testing could have been easily carried out but that it was not easily available was evidently a source of frustration. The general view in the meeting was that parents should have access to testing and then should be allowed to decide how best to proceed in the light of the information given. One participant said that he really did not know what he and his wife would have done with the results of a test. In a way that suggested the therapeutic gap might be narrowed, he pointed out that, as committed Christians, he and his wife would probably not have sought a termination, but the information would nonetheless have been helpful in enabling them to prepare for life with a child with a significant learning disability. This view was echoed by another participant, who said that if he had known what was to come he would have put money to one side to meet special needs and also have begun to find out about specialist services. Nobody in the meeting advocated termination, but the sentiment was clear: this should be a choice available to others.

An important theme in these discussions was that of mitigating disadvantage in the future. Significantly, this was not just about the child but, as the title of the PAASP clearly flags, the parents of the 'special child'. Parents of a child with Down's syndrome face economic hardship and distress which often leave the family, and particularly the mother, isolated. Indeed, in several instances, women interviewed had been deserted by their husbands following the birth of the child. This pattern was confirmed by the father of a boy with Down's syndrome who was active in an NGO providing children's homes for orphans of the war in the north and east. He described how fathers would often move away from the family as the child got older, leaving their wives in very precarious circumstances and resulting in the children being placed into care. This often left them being cared for alongside orphans created by the war.

Economic hardship is not the only concern, however. For many of the parents with whom I spoke, there were significant anxieties about the social impact that having a child with Down's syndrome would have on the family. In a society in which a high premium is placed on kinship and the extension of relations through marriage, the arrival of a child with serious learning disabilities is a major social catastrophe. In discussion with parents, it was clearly distressing for them to contemplate the fact that their child would probably never marry and reproduce. In one conversation, the woman was moved to tears at the thought of her son with Down's syndrome being 'alone' in later life. It was also a concern for parents that such a child could impede the marriage prospects of his or her siblings. The discovery that a future marriage partner had a sibling with learning difficulties could result in prospective relations being vetoed by parents and family. Several stories were related of families that had attempted to conceal the existence of a family member with learning difficulties only to have this discovered later and with serious consequences for interfamily relations.

Despite the strong feelings about the need to test expressed in this meeting and in other conversations with the parents of children with Down's syndrome, the question of acting on results and seeking a termination is approached with deep ambivalence. Unlike Deok et al (2002), however, who reported that a significant proportion of mothers seeking abortion felt that it should not be made easier for mothers to seek abortion, there was clear advocacy of the right for others to choose this course of action. This was partly an acknowledgement that, as relatively well off, middle-class families from Colombo, PAASP activists had mostly been in good positions to manage the arrival of a child with Down's syndrome constructively. However, there was acute awareness of the catastrophe that the arrival of a child with learning disabilities would have for the majority of less well off parents in Sri Lanka, and the massive social and economic risks that would ensue. Consequently, they were at pains to avoid dictating on moral, or indeed any other, grounds how families should respond when confronted with the knowledge that a child in utero would have significant disabilities. In other words, they were keen to promote reproductive freedom, but not in the abstract. Opting to produce children with major social disadvantages, who would in turn have an impact on wider networks of family and kin, is about more than simple parental preference. As Leach-Scully, Banks and Shakespeare (2006) have illustrated in relation to lay decision-making and prenatal sex selection in the UK, autonomous decision-making is an alien concept when it discounts the complex relational calculus that goes on when parents face difficult reproductive challenges. Decision-making is affected as much by concern about future persons and the web of relationships into which they will grow, as it is about choices made in the name of individual liberty and autonomy (also see Mackenzie and Stoljar 2000).

Later in the PAASP meeting, discussion of tests and the need for an early diagnosis began to turn to a contrasting set of concerns: not only were parents not able to get access to tests to find out at an early stage about their child's condition, but it also took them a long time to establish definitively the nature of their child's condition. Stories were shared as to how diagnoses were not confirmed until months after the child was born, despite all the signs being there from the outset. As in discussions with other parents of children with Down's syndrome, a view seemed to have been formed that doctors did not like to give bad news, and would rather refer the child on to another specialist than have to be the one giving a diagnosis. Prior to a definitive diagnosis, there was likely to have been a painful period in which parents had struggled to frame the meaning of what had befallen them. A combination of facial and bodily characteristics and a catalogue of health problems suggest to parents that a child has a serious problem, but ambiguous and partial messages from doctors and, indeed, the parents' own sense of denial about the child's condition, left them in a kind of limbo.

In conversation with other parents of children with Down's syndrome, it was clear that this limbo was not a time of inactivity, but one in which they were apt to draw on a range of other explanatory systems to account for the child's condition. As already suggested, for Sinhala Buddhists, explanations of how things come to pass invariably refer back to *karma*, the ultimate chain of actions and their consequences within which all suffering might be located. However, to invoke *karma* as an ultimate cause is not to eliminate the possibility that actions might be taken to maximise protection and mitigate the severity of what looks likely to come.

Faced with the unfolding tragedy of a child born with severe physical and mental disabilities, many parents initiated ritual activities, which they believed would complement straightforward biomedical interventions. For example, one Buddhist couple interviewed took the horoscope of their son to an astrologer shortly after it was realised that he had a congenital problem. The astrologer was quick to point out that the child was born in an inauspicious period governed by the planet Saturn and which would last for nine years (*senasuru erāstaka*). As a result of this prognosis, the couple undertook a wide range of ritual measures to mitigate the malign effects of the planet Saturn. They made regular offerings to the Buddha (*bodhi pujā*), they tied protective charms round the child's neck and arms (*yantra*), made vows at Hindu temples and said prayers at Christian churches. In their view, without this sustained and wide-ranging appeal to the benevolent powers of various religions, key developments, such as beginning to walk at the age of five, would not have happened. As with many couples faced with a major birth calamity, a consultation with an astrologer provides the beginnings of a meaningful narrative; it gives some explanation as to why things have happened as they have and, furthermore, indicates where their energies might be focused in order to protect the child in the light of its palpably inauspicious beginnings. Indeed, in certain respects, it could be argued that in astrology and the window it opens up on causality and fate, there are strong parallels with geneticists' notions of predisposition and susceptibility. Put simply, the astrologer's and the geneticist's interventions both offer their clients the prospect of future knowledge. However, in neither case is this knowledge hard in the sense of being absolute; it is hedged in language of chance and contingency. It also offers the possibility of being prepared for what might yet come to pass. Prenatal diagnostic testing yields a more dangerous knowledge. Once known, the intimations of the future that are found in chromosomes and genes cannot be un-known and, furthermore, once known give rise to some of the most challenging ethical dilemmas imaginable. The widespread belief, particularly among Buddhists and evidenced in beliefs in karmic consequences and the popularity of astrology, that the future can be known and anticipated through signs that are available in the present, is crucial in understanding the form that these dilemmas take. Genes, as a form of karmic inscription revealed by diagnostic testing, are likely to be given a particular place in attempts to make sense of misfortune.

However, the relationship between these different forms of knowledge is complex. A seriously muted response towards testing among public sector doctors needs to be contrasted with a burgeoning private sector ready to respond to market demand. Part of this demand is fuelled by an easy acceptance in Sri Lankan society of various kinds of determinism which are believed to underpin ideas of suffering and misfortune. The desire to know just where one lies in the *karmic* lottery and what actions might best bring security in an increasingly uncertain world manifest in a penchant for prediction which spans religious, ritual and biomedical systems. The availability of genetic testing kits, which are cheap and apparently easy to use, are proving to be a logical addition to the repertoire of tests that might be made available in the private sector to assist people in their desire to understand how the past has shaped the present and what this in turn means for the future. Given the social and economic costs that come with parenting children with a chronic illness, disability or learning difficulty on the one hand, and the relative ease of access to abortion on the other, it is hard to imagine that the option of termination would not begin to contribute in some small way to the current volume of terminations taking place in the island.

Some consequences of the therapeutic gap

By way of conclusion, I highlight some of the consequences of a failure to address the nature of the 'therapeutic gap' in the Sri Lankan context. There are issues of profound ethical significance to be found within the 'gap', and in what follows I offer some points of departure for future debate and research rather than definitive pronouncements. First, as things stand now, discussions regarding the ethics of prenatal genetic testing cannot take place in any meaningful way in the public sphere given the current disconnect between testing and termination. The possibility is thus raised that, without interventions that work within accepted professional guidelines, terminations might be triggered as a result of diagnoses obtained outside of well-regulated clinics and health services. As in other countries, unregulated prenatal diagnosis raises the prospect of termination taking place not only in the case of serious genetic disorders, but in relation to treatable conditions such as haemochromatosis or in response to parental preference, such as in prenatal sex selection. Moreover, it may be that decisions about termination are being made following testing undertaken in the private sector, which are not accompanied by any significant counselling or follow-up support. Second, the disconnection between testing and termination means that larger-scale issues of resource allocation cannot be addressed. For example, absence of effective screening for thalassaemia and the fact that more people affected by the disease can survive beyond childhood means that a major resource issue arises for the state in terms of provision of ongoing and regular blood transfusion and chelation therapy (De Silva et al 2000). Finally, in Sri Lanka today, the breadth of the 'therapeutic gap' is most acutely felt by parents themselves. The absence of information and therapeutic options leaves parents who are known to be carrying a child with severe genetic defects in a very difficult and desperate situation. They may be keen to narrow the 'therapeutic gap' on their own terms, that is, by anticipating the likely practical and financial consequences. Unfortunately, the harsh reality for many parents bringing up children with a chronic genetic condition is one of isolation, stigmatisation and hardship. The absence of appropriately conducted testing and access to open, professional and patient-focused counselling leaves couples abandoned to a fate which many believe they have brought upon themselves by their actions in a previous life. It is hardly surprising, therefore, that parents find their own ways of bridging the therapeutic divide, either by resorting to illegal abortion or by drawing on a range of non-medical beliefs and practices which help make sense of present events and give hope of ameliorating their likely future consequences.

Acknowledgements

I would like to express my sincere thanks to Dr Vajira Dissanayake, Professor Rohan Jayasekera and Mr Daksita Wickremasinghe for their help and cooperation in the conduct of the surveys referred to in this paper and their role in developing some of the ideas therein. Dr Prasanna Cooray provided invaluable assistance with the collection and transcription of interview data from some of the parents of children with Down's syndrome. The analysis and conclusions, however, remain entirely my own.

Notes

1   An interesting exception is to be found in Italy prior to 2003, where there was no state regulation of PGD, a thriving private sector market in reproductive services and a routine linkage between IVF and PGD, a soaring abortion rate, yet all against a backdrop of an overtly conservative attitude to abortion and the family (See www.tab.fzk.de/en/projekt/zusammenfassung/ab94.htm [Accessed 7 Oct 2009]; also see Bonnacorso 2004.)
2   I followed the activities of the PAASP for a period of three months. Interviews were also carried out with twelve parents of children with Down's syndrome. Some of these were members of PAASP and others were recruited through community contacts.

3   Private and Public Eugenics

Genetic Testing and Screening in India

Jyotsna Agnihotri Gupta

Genetic testing and eugenics

Epidemiologists and geneticists claim that genetics has an increasing role to play in public health policies and programmes in the future. Within this perspective, genetic testing and screening are instrumental in avoiding the birth of children with serious, costly or untreatable disorders. There is a globalisation of testing and screening technologies in countries with very diverse health systems and services, socio-economic conditions within which users and service providers operate, and ethical and legal institutions responsible for overseeing practices. Reproductive genetics is one field in which the development and application of technology is proliferating very rapidly in developing countries, including India. We can expect that the use of genetic testing technology will have serious and far-reaching implications for cultural perceptions regarding health and disease and women's experience of pregnancy, besides creating new ethical dilemmas and new professional and parental responsibilities.

The primary goal of genetic testing and screening is to provide information that helps pregnant women/couples to take their own reproductive decisions, not to reduce the number of genetic diseases in the population. Though norms may differ, the desire to have a healthy and normal baby is universal. Every pregnant woman/couple/family wants a good reproductive outcome and the state wants a healthy population; in this sense they share a common goal. While some believe that genetic testing offers new possibilities for informed decision-making to (prospective) parents and consumers, others fear social pressure, marginalisation and stigmatisation and some form of eugenics as a consequence of its application.

The term 'eugenics' comes from the Greek *eugenes* for 'good birth'. It was first used by Francis Galton, a cousin of Darwin, in 1883 with the publication of his book *Inquiries into Human Faculty and its Development*, to mean 'healthy birth'. Eugenics emerged as an extension of the science of heredity, and it claims to apply genetic principles for the improvement of 'mankind'. There are two kinds of eugenics: positive and negative. Positive eugenics aims to increase the reproduction of 'fit' individuals; negative eugenics aims to reduce the reproduction of 'unfit' individuals. Recent developments in basic genomics research may be eugenic in nature, in that 'the aim is not only to "cure" disease – it is also to alter the genetic make-up of animals and humans, to get rid of "bad" genes from the population. In the language of eugenics, it is to promote the reproduction of fit individuals' (Ewing 1988: 34). Ewing noted that the increased emphasis on looking for genetic causes of disease, while neglecting social and environmental factors, can be likened to the theories of socio-biology and biological determinism.

Wertz et al (2003: 10) define eugenics as '[a] coercive policy intended to further a reproductive goal, against the rights, freedoms, and choices of the individual'. They argue that 'eugenics is directed against whole populations, whereas the work of today's clinical geneticists is directed towards individuals and families.' They find little evidence for eugenic practice in the modern world. American bioethicist Kitcher (1996) suggests that some form of eugenics is inevitable, and that it is acceptable provided it is voluntary and practised on an individual basis without social coercion. The 'utopian eugenics' that Kitcher envisages would attempt a fine balance between 'compassionate abortion' (after prenatal diagnosis of severely disabling conditions and a very restricted future life) and enabling services for future disabled people with even the most severe medical conditions.

Agar (2004), using the concept of 'liberal eugenics', argues for giving a choice to individuals to use reproductive and genetic technologies to enhance their children's genetic opportunities. This term is used to differentiate it from the collectivist, authoritarian and totalitarian eugenic programmes of the first half of the twentieth century. The idea is to allow parents to exercise procreative liberty both to minimise congenital disorders and to enhance desired capacities in their children. Agar uses the classical Rawlsian liberal theory to justify eugenic freedom, like other liberal freedoms, in the context of the recent scientific developments in the field of genetics, as well as the discourse surrounding these technological developments in terms of individualism and the market economy. Since liberal eugenics relies on new reprogenetic technologies, it is often referred to as 'neo-eugenics' or 'techno-eugenics'. Because of its individual and market orientation, it is sometimes also termed 'consumer eugenics'. Two contrasting stereotypes permeate the media coverage of genetics: 'genetic optimism', a sense that genetic discoveries will 'revolutionise the diagnosis, prevention and treatment' of human diseases, and the 'discourse of concern', a view infused with fear towards genetic technologies and ethical concerns emerging from it (Catz et al 2005: 162).

The most important opposition to the research and application of gene technology is based on the fear of a return of (positive and negative) eugenics, as practised in the early twentieth century in the US, and up until the 1970s in several European countries. Positive and negative eugenics ideas are still expressed openly and also practised, either covertly or openly, both in the West and in several Asian countries, including India, China, Japan and Singapore. This may take the form of open or veiled coercion to undergo genetic testing or screening for hereditary or congenital disorders, followed (in the case of prenatal screening) by abortion or sterilisation.

This chapter is based on a literature review and empirical research using qualitative methods, which included participant observation in genetic and ultrasound clinics and the thalassaemia unit of a private trust hospital in New Delhi. This was followed by individual interviews with service providers and some of the counselled women/couples. In the case of thalassaemia, besides service providers, parents of thalassaemic children were interviewed.

In this chapter, I use the term 'eugenics' in its original sense of 'healthy birth' and I distinguish 'private' from 'public' eugenics. I refer to the practice of prenatal diagnosis as an aspect of private eugenics when the initiative to test comes from the pregnant woman herself. Public eugenics involves testing initiated by the state or medical profession and medical institutions, through testing programmes, which may be more or less obligatory. I argue that in some cases there appears to be only a thin line distinguishing individual choice and overt or covert coercion, and between 'private' and 'public' eugenics. To illustrate these concepts, I discuss the management of thalassaemia, which I see as an example of private eugenics that is moving into the sphere of public eugenics. I then discuss the recently launched newborn screening programme as an example of public eugenics. Foucault's theory and concepts of 'power' and 'governmentality' are used to explore the thin line separating individual choice and overt or covert coercion, and between 'private' and 'public' eugenics.

Genomics for health in India

Curbing the population growth rate and size remains the main objective of health and family welfare programmes in India; controlling the quality of the human gene pool does not seem to be a stated priority of the state. This may change once stabilisation of the population is achieved. Both the central and state governments have made substantial investments in biomedical research in order to tackle India's unmet medical needs and to improve the overall health of the population (Kumar et al 2004). According to India's Department of Biotechnology (DBT), sixteen genetic diagnosis and counselling units have been set up in India for prenatal diagnosis and counselling for major genetic disorders (www.dbtindia.nic.in). Human cytogenetics (the study of chromosomes and related diseases) for disorders other than cancer is conducted at the All India Institute of Medical Sciences (AIIMS) and Department of Genetic Medicine, Sir Ganga Ram Hospital in Delhi, KEM Hospital Mumbai, St John Medical College, Bangalore, and some centres in Pune. Besides these, there are nine other units in private hospitals, bringing the total number to 25 (personal communication, Dr I.C. Verma, genetic counsellor).

While genetic testing and screening programmes are becoming more or less routine in many countries in the West, in most developing countries like India the public health[1] exchequer is unable to bear the costs of large-scale programmes; thus it is left largely to the private health sector to offer the services. In general, public-sector hospitals lack financial resources to meet the huge demand for genetic testing and counselling from patients who often cannot afford to pay the charges at private hospitals/clinics.

The most common indication for seeking genetic counselling is reproductive genetics, of which prenatal diagnosis is the most common. According to the Indian Society for Prenatal Diagnosis and Therapy (IS-PAT), which held its eighth national conference in New Delhi on 17-19 February 2006, over 25 million births take place in India annually; 16 million babies suffer from some kind of disorder. Cytogenetic abnormalities may be responsible for early embryonic death, minor to major congenital defects, infertility or sterility, as well as cancer. Genetic testing and counselling is underdeveloped in India. Those seeking genetic counselling and prenatal diagnosis (PND) are mainly couples with a family history of a particular disease, parents of children who already have an affected child, or women with a history of repeated miscarriages due to advanced maternal age. Counselling and PND are sought on the advice of family, friends, a family doctor, gynaecologist, or paediatrician. Prenatal tests are not offered routinely to pregnant women, but are becoming common in large cities as pregnant women are increasingly registering with gynaecologists for antenatal care and delivery in clinics rather than having traditional home births, although the latter is still the norm in rural areas, where the majority of the population lives. PND for monitoring fetal growth and development through ultrasound and certain blood tests may indicate a higher risk of genetic or congenital abnormalities. Preimplantation genetic diagnosis (PGD) of the embryo is also becoming a more common adjunct to assisted reproduction using IVF, which is itself proliferating at a fast pace. Genetic screening of newborns is gradually being introduced in certain selected centres. Given the paucity of institutional facilities for the disabled, and the financial and care burden this brings for families with a child who is either disabled, or suffers from a genetic condition, there is an increasing demand for genetic testing services and genetic counselling.

The most common genetic disorders in India are Down's syndrome, thalassaemia, Duchenne muscular dystrophy, spinal muscular atrophy, and inborn errors of metabolism. Thalassaemia is one of the conditions where we can observe the convergence of 'private' and 'public' eugenics – that is, testing being offered as individual choice, although initiated by the medical profession and hospital policy in some cases.

Thalassaemia

Thalassaemia is the most common single-gene disorder. It affects over 30 million people worldwide. Only 3 per cent of the population in India carries it. Although this is low compared to Cyprus, where the corresponding figure is 15 per cent, the absolute numbers of affected individuals in India are high, due to its large population. Thalassaemia is more common in certain parts of India and among certain communities, such as Punjabis, Sindhis, Gujaratis, Gaurs, Marwaris and Saraswats. It is less prevalent in south India.

Every year, between 7,000 and 10,000 children are born with thalassaemia major in India. They survive on periodic blood transfusions and chelation therapy, which is very expensive. The medical costs for a child suffering from this disorder can be around 10,000 rupees[2] a month (approximately US $ 235: note that India's average per capita income is only about US $ 820).

The only cure for thalassaemia is bone marrow transplantation, which few can afford. The life expectancy of those affected is between 20 and 35 years. Facilities for treatment are neither available nor accessible in most parts of the country. Thalassaemia is considered preventable if prospective parents are tested, and all pregnant women are tested in early pregnancy for thalassaemia status and undergo abortion if the foetus is affected.

I conducted interviews with parents of thalassaemic children and with Dr V. K. Khanna, a paediatrician with a special interest in thalassaemia. He founded the thalassaemia unit at Sir Ganga Ram Hospital (SGRH) twenty years ago, and is Vice President of Thalassemics India. According to Dr Khanna, most couples come for the thalassaemia test as part of antenatal testing. Only occasionally do individuals come for a premarital thalassaemia test. As Dr Khanna explained:

I do not counsel premarital thalassaemia. If they come to know that the prospective bride or groom is a carrier, no one will marry a person with thalassaemia minor. There is so much interference from parents and grandparents. They must be told that individuals with thalassaemia minor are normal people.

In the social climate of India, knowledge of someone's thalassaemic status can be stigmatising for the individual. Dr Khanna clarified: 'In a university in Gujarat, they asked for thalassaemia status on the admission form; but there was such a hue and cry that they stopped, because there is no law that you must have a blood test.'

During interviews, most parents mentioned to me that they had not even heard of the disease called thalassaemia before the birth of their affected child. Many parents reported that they had first sought treatment for their child from practitioners of traditional (Aryuvedic) medicine and homeopathy. As a mother (RD) of a thalassaemic son put it:

We didn't even think that we would have this problem, because my husband and I were apparently normal. We were going for homeopathic and Aryuvedic treatment for his height problem, as he was not growing well. ... Every couple should be told about thalassaemia after marriage, in fact before marriage; if both are thalassaemic, they should not marry.

Most large hospitals in big Indian cities are now doing thalassaemia tests routinely on all pregnant women as part of antenatal check-ups and on every child that is born. Dr Khanna related, 'In SGRH all our children are thalassaemia-free. All [pregnant] women go for antenatal diagnosis and abort in case the foetus is affected. Because if it is in the family, they have seen the hardship, and trauma and the cost, so they immediately opt for the test'.

In the words of another mother (AM):

Now, testing is compulsory at SGRH, but it should be made compulsory everywhere. Not only does the child suffer, but the whole family suffers. In our family we tell the others to get the test done, but they think we must have some personal interest in it, so they don't listen. They should get the test done premaritally, or just after marriage.

In 1996, the Delhi government introduced the thalassaemia prevention programme in all Delhi administration (public) hospitals. All pregnant women undergo the test. By and large, all private hospitals and some private gynaecologists also conduct the test. An earlier study showed that the affected foetus is generally aborted (Thakore 1994). Dr Khanna explained:

> Only once I had a woman who had conceived after a long time. The gynaecologist advised prenatal testing, but her in-laws didn't accept. They put pressure on her to continue the pregnancy. She produced a thalassaemia major child.

In India, the expenditure incurred by parents/families of thalassaemic children is prohibitive. In many cases patients and their families must travel long distances – inter-state even – as the facilities for treatment and blood transfusion are available only in a few metropolitan centres. Dr Khanna explained:

> The costs are 550 rupees per transfusion. Costs may be less of a barrier at SGRH, because here we deal with the cream of society. But, if you look at the overall picture in the country, more than 95 per cent people can't afford it. The pump costs 10,000-12,000 rupees and each vial of Desferal costs 175-180 rupees. It comes up to 15-20,000 rupees a month. We are helping poor patients by raising funds for them. During general OPD [outpatients department] clinic hours I do tests and check-ups at 50 per cent less charges and free counselling.

Private health insurance, which very few can afford, does not cover the cost of thalassaemia care or any related problem; only some employees of large government undertakings or multinational/private companies are able to get compensation for costs incurred. As one mother (RD) said, 'Please write this down. At AIIMS [All India Institute of Medical Sciences, a public hospital] we got no attention, but everybody cannot afford to come to SGRH.' Another mother (RA) said, 'On the whole what we earn is for the child. We have no savings.'

When I asked whether women are blamed for producing a thalassaemic child, Dr Khanna answered in the negative, and so did most mothers and fathers of thalassaemic children. However, one woman (RA) had this to say:

> My father-in-law said my son got the disease from his nani's [maternal grandmother's] house. Do the nana-nani [maternal grandparents] wish bad things for their grandchild? They would rather wish the best. In some families they say the woman has brought the disease from her mother's house. In 90 per cent cases the woman is blamed. The woman is underpowered in the household.

Mrs S. Tuli, Secretary of Thalassemics India, also agrees that women are blamed. 'Here, most people think the daughter-in-law is to be blamed. ... Most parents think their son is perfectly healthy.'

Also, the prejudice against girl children leading to their prebirth elimination in India could be further aggravated in the case of children affected by thalassaemia. According to a gynaecologist/obstetrician (Dr PB):

> They will abort a thalassaemic girl; if it's a boy they will continue the pregnancy. We come to know because they don't even come to pick up the report. The sad thing in this country is that the doctors themselves are stakeholders in the abortion of female foetuses.

In my opinion, the gender aspects of thalassaemia clearly need to be explored further.

In conjunction with carrier screening, prenatal diagnosis and termination of the affected foetus can reduce the prevalence of thalassaemia:

> Treatment of thalassaemia is expensive, arduous and painful. It is associated with complications of chelation therapy, and the risk of transfusion-related infections. It is, therefore, necessary to prevent the birth of affected children by prenatal diagnosis, to reduce the socio-economic pressure on the family and the burden of disease on the community. Therefore, genetic counselling and prenatal diagnosis (PND) are essential to control this dreaded disease. (Saxena 2006)

In the words of a mother (RD): 'They should give information on thalassaemia in the media – on TV and in the news. There is attention in the media for cancer and HIV/AIDS, but not for thalassaemia.' A father (PA) strongly urged:

> There should be a campaign to publicise that thalassaemia is even more serious than AIDS, and it comes from the parents. Gynaecologists should test routinely for thalassaemia. Nobody is doing anything about it or publicising this. Also, there is no public or state support for those affected.

Dr Khanna gives lectures to the Delhi Gynaecological Society urging that it should be offered as a routine test. Mrs S. Tuli emphasised:

> We say 'get yourself tested before marriage, as students, or after marriage before planning your family. ...' You have to screen fa-

milies. Families should test their other children. They have some responsibility towards the country. The ideal in this respect are Cyprus and Italy. ... There has to be a campaign by the government; big names must be involved in the publicity. The message should be that it is a genetic problem and must be controlled. Thalassaemia patients use so much blood, which is difficult to obtain, which could be used for other needy patients. All the medicines – needle (infusion set), pump and Desferal are imported. We could save on foreign exchange. The money that goes to the NGOs could be saved. Most patients, if they do not have the financial means, die early and do not contribute to society because of this disease. The ideal way is to prevent it, and it is preventable. We have to educate the people. The government has to earmark funds for it. Thalassaemia can be eradicated.

From the quotes above, which voice individual parental desires regarding avoiding the birth of thalassaemic children and medical specialists' views urging the importance of thalassemia testing and offering testing services to pregnant women, we can see how *private* and *public* eugenics converge.

Genetic screening is accorded an even more important role in public health through the practice of newborn screening. I will now examine the relevance of this practice for public health in India.

Newborn screening

Screening programmes target the wider population in order to identify individuals who are at risk of having children with genetic disorders. Guidelines adopted in various developed countries state the importance of screening all newborns before they leave the hospital for certain endocrinopathies, metabolic errors and hearing loss. Newborn infants are screened for congenital metabolic variations needing immediate intervention to prevent the progression of disease. Screening is thus conducted with the goals of both primary prevention (i.e. to identify the risk of disease and intervene so as to avoid it entirely) and secondary prevention (i.e. to intervene medically so as to mitigate the consequences of disease and improve the prognosis for patients).

In most countries of the developed West, newborn screening for treatable Mendelian disorders has been provided under public health programmes since the 1960s. Screening was first applied for phenylketonuria (PKU). Screening of newborns has become a routine and often mandatory procedure, and is often subsidised by the government, although the number of conditions for which screening occurs may vary across countries. Conditions such as PKU, haemoglobinopathies, e.g. sickle-cell disease, congenital hypothyroidism (CH), congenital adrenal hyperplasia (CAH), cystic fibrosis (CF) and intrauterine infections such as toxoplasmosis and deafness, are generally part of regular screening programmes. Parents may opt out on religious or other grounds, although often they are not informed about this possibility.

The range of disorders for which newborns can be screened has increased with the use of tandem mass spectrometry (TMS) and DNA testing. With the help of TMS about 30 metabolic genetic disorders can be detected from one sample, and the diagnosis is available in one day. This technology can detect the presence of disorders before the appearance of clinical symptoms, providing enough time to save the child from mental retardation, early death and other physical disabilities (Lal & Kaur 2006). However, the technology is expensive, and even in the US some states cannot afford it, particularly in times of budget deficits (Holtzman 2006).

About 5 per cent of all pregnancies result in the birth of a child with a significant genetic disorder, congenital malformation or disability (Wertz et al 2003). In India, over 25 million births occur annually. The infant and child mortality rate is very high, and infectious diseases are still the primary cause. Geneticists argue, however, that India is undergoing an epidemiological transition: many neonatal infections are better controlled today, which means that over time, the proportion of perinatal mortality attributable to birth defects has increased. If the incidence of birth defects is assumed to be 2 per cent, then 500,000 babies are born with some form of birth defect every year in India (Verma & Bijarnia 2002). Paediatricians argue that prevention is the best strategy, given that cure after birth is difficult and costly.

According to geneticists, the incidence of metabolic disorders is on the increase in India. An estimated 9,760 infants are born with amino acid disorders each year (Verma & Bijarnia 2002); UNICEF (2004) estimates are even higher – 12,500 children annually. If this is not detected early enough, in most cases this leads to irreversible brain damage as time progresses. 'That some infants aren't being caught and treated when possible is a national tragedy and TMS should be standard care for all newborns, much as blood pressure test is a part of every medical check-up' (Hanon 2004). Some geneticists argue in favour of neonatal karyotyping (chromosomal fingerprinting) of all newborns. In India, this would be an impossible task, as the majority of births take place at home and the infrastructure and facilities for genetic testing are poor and too few. An ideal time for collection of samples is from the third to the seventh day after birth; this is not feasible in most hospitals, where the delivery rate is very high and early discharge policies are in place.

Unlike many Western countries, neonatal screening is still not routine in India. Generally, only high-risk newborns and infants are screened. This happens usually after obstetricians/gynaecologists advise parents to consult other specialists such as neonatologists, paediatricians, neurologists and geneticists. There are only two pilot studies which have been conducted for comprehensive screening of neonates. The first was in Bangalore in 1980, to calculate the incidence of amino acid disorders. A second pilot programme, the Expanded Newborn Screening, was started in Hyderabad in 2000.[3] These pilot studies established a high prevalence of inherited metabolic disease in Indian newborns and highlighted the importance of initiating multicentre testing for the common disorders throughout the country.

Recently, the Indian Council for Medical Research (ICMR) invited proposals to set up centres in different parts of the country, to screen newborns at several centres in India to assess the kind of genetic defects they develop. This initiative aims to diagnose affected children at an early age in order to improve possibilities for treatment of genetic and metabolic defects before they develop into life-long burdens.

Another important rationale for screening is to find out the prevalence of the types of genetic conditions in the Indian population. All newborns will be screened within three to four days of birth by means of blood and urine diagnostic tests so that, if necessary, treatment can begin three weeks after delivery, which is believed to be more effective than when it occurs at a later age. It is seen as a public health measure in terms of primary and secondary prevention, leading to a significant reduction in morbidity, mortality and disabilities, and to improved health. Since the programme is to be launched as an experiment, it has been agreed to limit screening only for two conditions – congenital hypothyroidism (leading to mental retardation, developmental delay) and congenital adrenal hyperplasia (diarrhoea, dehydration, ambiguous genitalia) – in order to be able to offer ethical treatment, management and counselling [Dr Roli Mathur, scientist, ICMR, personal communication]. When I asked whether it can lead to stigmatisation of the child or its family, Dr Ratna, [geneticist at SGRH, personal communication] replied: 'Not at all. If undiagnosed, it might be a severe presentation later. These are diseases that are treatable through medicines.'

Neonatal screening is already being conducted at several hospitals. The first expanded programme was initiated in Hyderabad in 2000 to screen all newborns in four major government maternity hospitals (Newborn Screener 2005). The program currently includes testing for congenital adrenal hyperplasia, hypothyroidism and G6PD (an enzyme deficiency causing sensitivity to certain drugs) and may be extended later to detect other disorders which include, besides amino acid disorders, biotinidase deficiency and galactosaemia. Samples are taken before infants are discharged from hospital. The baby's birth weight is registered and the parents are informed of the test results. The screening programme is not truly voluntary but implemented as 'routine without notification'. In other words, medical personnel take the consent of parents for granted, or as tacitly given, either when the baby is born in the hospital/clinic, or later when they seek neonatal medical care. Quite often the parents do not even know that the testing will be performed. It is subsumed, conceptually as well as procedurally, under routine neonatal care, and ceases to be something about which a deliberate decision has to be made by the parents. As contended by van den Daele (2006: 43):

> This practice thus amounts to de facto mandatory genetic screening; nevertheless, it goes virtually unchallenged, which is evidence that, despite official tribute to the principle of informed consent, coercive strategies may prevail to ensure that the preventive benefits of genetic screening can be reaped.

However, this should not be the case. As Holtzman (2006:12) notes:

> Unless they are compulsory, genetic services are active strategies, requiring the acquiescence of individuals. In most places newborn screening is mandatory, but it is not a passive strategy because parental compliance is needed if screening is to prevent disabilities.

While many conditions may be diagnosed by screening, there is a lack of effective treatment for most of them. This 'therapeutic gap' (Holtzman & Shapiro 1998) begs an important question: if there is no effective treatment available, what is the value of testing? Treatment options should be in place before at-risk populations are identified by screening tests. In India, parents may not be able to distinguish between screening and treatment, and may cherish false hopes that after screening the child will automatically receive treatment and become healthy, or at least free of the disease for which she or he was screened. Where treatments exist, many parents are unlikely to be able to afford the high costs of ongoing treatment.

In order to prevent birth defects, and provide supportive care for the affected, it is essential to know the incidence and prevalence of birth defects in India. Although there are some statistics available from several hospital-based studies, it is difficult to generalise these to the wider population due to selection biases. Geneticists and paediatricians argue that an active birth defects registry will rectify this. Hence, The Fetal Care Research Foundation, a not-for-profit charitable trust, founded the

Birth Defects Registry of India in Chennai in 2001. More centres are expected to be set up in other parts of the country in the near future. The data collected by the registries will help the government formulate plans and build strategies to combat the problem of birth defects. It will also provide clinicians and consultants with accurate information to pass on to parents during counselling.

There are some ethical issues related to newborn screening that need attention.

> Newborn screening would seem to be the antithesis of eugenics. Saving life and improving its quality rather than avoiding the birth of infants with serious genetic diseases is the primary goal of newborn screening. However, in a recent US survey of 'follow-up coordinators' of newborn screening programmes, the respondents in 19 states thought that children identified by newborn screening were 'unsuitable choices for future reproduction' and that conveying this information should be one of the goals of counselling their parents. (Holtzman 2006: 14)

In this way, a new class of 'unpatients' is created, even though the disease may not even have manifested itself (Jonsen et al 1996).

An even more important ethical concern is how to ensure confidentiality, and prevent stigmatisation and discrimination of affected children and their families, who may be viewed as genetically 'abnormal'. In the Indian cultural context, newborn screening may exacerbate the problem of finding a marriage partner, especially if the 'affected' child is female. It may result in individuals and families becoming social outcasts, this time not on, or not only on, the basis of (low) caste affiliation, but also on genetic grounds. The Department of Biotechnology website (op. cit) mentions that a few thousand people belonging to socially underprivileged groups, including those from Scheduled Castes (SCs) and Scheduled Tribes (STs), have been screened for various genetic disorders. While the prevalence of sickle-cell anaemia is highest in tribal populations, these groups may have been singled out due to eugenic anxieties that are common both among the general public and among policy makers, viz. that higher castes and economically privileged groups are producing fewer children, and those from the lower castes and the poorer sections of society are responsible for most population growth.

The health insurance industry in India is still in a nascent stage, but it is expanding. Insurers may use information about positive test results to limit their own risks at the expense of those who have undergone the tests and been found to be at 'risk'. Genetic traits that lead to disease are literally 'embodied risks'. 'This discourse of risk implicates these practices and procedures in relations of power in ways that, for the most part, have not been critically interrogated' (Tremain 2006: 37).

> Public health policies that focus on individual risk factors are met with suspicion because they could lead to 'blaming the victim' instead of striving for social change, and because they restrict individual freedom and place private choice under public surveillance. (Van den Daele 2006: 41)

Decision-making processes: the construction of choice

Although decision-making processes are often considered in bioethics from the point of view of the 'autonomous individual', choices are always prestructured by a range of factors including limited information and understanding, cultural values and beliefs, family attitudes and influence, faith and religion, and social and economic conditions. 'Informed choice' and 'informed decision-making' in the context of genetic testing entail at least that the decision should be based on relevant information regarding the characteristics of screening tests, and the implications of the possible test results. It also entails that the decision should be consistent with the decision-maker's values. Accepting or declining screening should be founded on informed choice, because of the risks and moral values that play a part. Prenatal screening may lead to diagnostic testing, which involves the risk of an iatrogenic abortion and, in case of a positive test result, to the option of terminating a pregnancy. Informed choice implies the ability or competence to understand complicated statistical relationships between genes and diseases. The goal of screening programmes should thus be to enable people to make informed choices, rather than achieve the maximum possible uptake rates.

International research has shown that often women/couples lack sufficient knowledge about the different aspects of (prenatal) screening, which impedes informed decision-making. Informed choice appears to be associated with the educational attainment of the pregnant woman/couple. Higher education levels correlate with higher levels of informed choice (van den Berg et al 2005). My own research corroborates this. The higher the education level of the couples I interviewed, the more they actively sought information from service providers, books and the Internet. This group expressed some measure of satisfaction regarding the genetic counselling they received, whereas women/couples with lower educational levels seemed less satisfied that they were getting enough information. This could have to do with the complexity of the information, and unfamiliarity with the language in which it was couched. The latter group tended to ask fewer questions during counselling sessions, and when I interviewed them thereafter they asked me questions, which they should have put to the counsellor. The gap between those able to handle this complexity and those who cannot will have the potential to be a new kind of social inequality (Brand 2005).

It is difficult to ascertain whether all decisions are the result of a process of deliberation. There is little information available on the role of the family in decision-making in India. My observation is that even where decisions ultimately fall to the couples and they do not feel under overt pressure from the family, the whole family is involved in the process of seeking help. One or more family members may accompany the pregnant woman/couple when she goes for prenatal tests, and participate in decision-making thereafter, especially if the couple lives in a joint or extended family setting. Sometimes, there appears to be a difference of opinion between the woman and her husband regarding the course to follow, especially if it is very expensive and involves recurring costs. Gender differences in attitudes towards genetic testing and decisions made thereafter should be explored further, especially given that women bear the main burden of responsibility for taking care of disabled children.

Informed choice also implies respect for the client's autonomy, which, like the concepts privacy and confidentiality, and patient rights, is an underdeveloped concept in the Indian cultural context. Indian patients rely heavily on the doctor's advice about what course of action should be followed, and because doctors are usually regarded with a high degree of reverence, patients seldom question their judgement. This poses problems for the principle of non-directive counselling and obtaining truly informed consent from women/couples for testing procedures. There are no indications that geneticists and genetic counsellors pursue a hidden public health agenda by talking parents into aborting pregnancies against their will in order to reduce the burden of congenital diseases in the population (Van den Daele 2006). The 'pressure' to choose abortion after PND is more subtle: it arises mainly from the parents' own understanding that it is 'not fair toward a child to bring it to birth with a severe disability'. This was the most common answer I received when I asked women whether they faced pressure in their decision-making process.

> Thus, while it seems inconceivable that it will ever be adopted in our societies as public policy or legal concept that parents who knowingly bring foetuses with severe handicaps to birth commit child abuse, parents may nevertheless feel pressure to terminate such pregnancies – pressure from social environments which

disagree and pressure from 'within' themselves in terms of moral doubt.   (Van den Daele 2006: 47)

Absence of manifest coercion must not be taken as proof that people
can take truly autonomous decisions. While individuals may feel that
they pursue their private preferences, they in fact execute collective
functions and comply with social controls that they have internalised.
Foucault's theory of power and his concept of 'governmentality' are useful to analyse the connections between power, medicine and reproduction in modern society. Foucault (1980, 1982, 1991) differentiates between juridical power, which is based on public rights, and the disciplinary power of the norm. He links the latter to the rise of a specific
medical/scientific discourse that was brought to bear on the body during the eighteenth and nineteenth centuries. This discourse emerged
alongside new medical practices and techniques, which were refined in
the emerging institution of the clinic. The totality of these developments gave rise to a new type of power, closely tied to the development
of a specific kind of knowledge.

According to Foucault, medical power is diffuse in character; it is to
be found everywhere and at the same time it is difficult to pinpoint. It
creates an order in society by 'normalising' (i.e. by differentiating between the normal and the abnormal). The normalising, disciplinary
power of medicine is inextricably tied to the development of advances
in medicine and medical knowledge, and medical institutions come to
play a central role in the moral regulation of the population.

The disciplinary power of the norm and the juridical power of laws
are closely intertwined. Foucault points out that one of the first effects
of medical politics is the restructuring and medicalisation of the family.
A whole system of medical care is built up around children, and the family bears the responsibility for this system of care, serving as a link
between the health of society as a general political objective and the individual need for healthcare. The power that accrues to those who are at
the top of the hierarchy of sex, race, caste, class – as embodied in the
person of the doctor – can be accounted for using a more traditional account of power as domination.

'Governmentality' assumes that, in modern societies, the locus of collective control is shifting from overt patterns of power and domination
to implicit orders represented in social and cultural discourses and
practices. According to this line of argument, power operates increasingly through self-regulation and self-discipline rather than violence or
domination:

[T]he 'order of the self', i.e. what people conceive as rational, morally binding and desirable, reproduces collective imperatives and

> social control. This reasoning reminds us that individual beliefs and preferences do not emerge from outside the society: rather they are acquired through the processes of socialisation and ac-culturation. (Van den Daele 2006: 48)

Individual choice is often used as an argument in favour of the expansion of genetic testing services. Most of the interventions take place in the area of reproductive genetics. There is a widespread view among clinicians, scientists and policy makers that the birth of a disabled child is a tragedy best avoided. Just as in the past, professionals are making decisions about what kind of people ought to be born, and these decisions have a profound effect on people undergoing genetic diagnosis and making the ultimate choice about whether or not to continue with their pregnancies. Professionals have an inordinate amount of power and control over what genetic research gets conducted, how genetics is applied in the clinic and beyond in the wider community, and how genetic research and services are regulated (Kerr & Shakespeare 2002).

There are degrees of coercion and different domains of control (van den Daele 2006: 42). Degrees of coercion may include direct or indirect legal force, conditions for access to institutions and services, economic incentives, persuasion and education, professional dominance, instilling a sense of moral duty and self-determination as societal governance. Domains of control could include mandatory newborn screening, routine screening (antenatal and postnatal) without notification, 'active' counselling of persons at risk and who want to know the risks in deference to the predominant cultural patterns of rationality. The concept of 'risk' has itself become a central organising principle of governmentality. Professional biases against handicapped children may be applied as pressure to abort through directive counselling. For parents, it may imply a sense of moral duty, accepting a responsibility to bring only healthy children to birth. 'Individual' preferences for a healthy child thus comply with fundamentally social norms.

Waldschmidt (1992: 164-165) refers to genetic testing and prenatal diagnosis as 'neo-eugenics' and 'the new grassroots eugenics'. Neo-eugenics does not need to operate through direct forms of coercion, pressure, open repression or control as part of government policy. The state and society no longer need to intervene in order to urge people to do their eugenic duty, because now people 'voluntarily' adhere to eugenic lines of reasoning individually, without being expressly told to do so. It is supported and practised 'from below'. The choice of the individual becomes the medium through which 'government is exercised' (Koch & Svendsen 2005: 824).

Most people agree that it is better to prevent disease than to cure it; they accept that they ought to participate in prevention out of duty to the community. Notions of rational behaviour, a sense of moral duty, and visions of a good life also shape individual preferences. As a result, people tend to bring about through their private choice what might otherwise be imposed on them through public policy. They even achieve as a collective effect of their individual choices the reduction of the prevalence of congenital diseases through selective abortion, which could not be legitimately pursued in public health programmes, because that would be read as a return to eugenic policy (Van den Daele 2006: 47-48). I see this being played out in decision-making processes during prenatal procedures in India.

Given the history of population control in India, the spectre of coercion still looms in India's public health policy. We may yet see the revival of state-driven mandatory preventive strategies, which turn genetic testing into a means of social control to enforce compliance with collective goals – and yet give the impression of having democratic support. Short of this, the tension between public health objectives and individual freedom will tend to remain invisible so long as there is widespread voluntary compliance with genetic testing and screening programmes.

The guidelines on human genetics formulated by the Indian Council of Medical Research (ICMR 2000) have been widely circulated among the medical community. The DBT has also adopted policies on ethics and regulatory issues in biotechnology. Principles of informed consent and confidentially are enshrined in them. However, in the absence of binding legislation and additional resources for monitoring, their implementation depends on the scientific community. 'There is no way that the ICMR can be the policing agency,' says Vasantha Mutthuswamy, chief of basic biomedical research at ICMR and secretary of the Central Ethics Committee on Human Research, which formulated the guidelines.

What is significant in this respect is the move towards privatisation of responsibility for health in neoliberal societies, accompanied by the promotion of particular choices. As Ann Kerr (2004: 82) points out, 'What is at stake today is a privatisation of responsibilities for preventing disability, or, if a test is declined, facing up to the future of living with a disabled child.' This process is not value-neutral: making individuals responsible for the birth of healthy infants is the product of a moral discourse, which is in part politically motivated, even if it appears entirely reasonable. It requires a commitment to shared social values and behavioural expectations on the part of both individuals and the societies they inhabit. With the proliferation of genetic tests, testing is becoming a part of 'good parenthood' at the individual level; at the societal level, community genetics is emerging as a practice and as a future model, in which the options offered by genetic screening technologies can be used optimally for the realisation of preventive healthcare. In this way, 'private' and 'public' eugenics merge.

Informed consent prior to screening would seem to negate any 'eugenic' connotation. Considering how programmes are conducted, however – the incomplete information often given to women/couples considering an antenatal screening, the financial and care burden of raising children with conditions for which screening is possible, and increasing intolerance in society for imperfection and failure to use prenatal diagnosis – the eugenic overtones are clear (Holtzman 2006: 14).

Other concerns related to genetic testing and screening in India

Is it ever justified to persuade or coerce people to undergo screening tests, either through government mandate or by exerting more subtle psychological pressures? Fear of genetic stigmatisation or discrimination may deprive people of the real benefits of early diagnosis, treatment or prevention that result from newborn screening. Unless there is a guarantee that test results and medical records are kept confidential, as well as protection of privacy for individuals and families and effective protection against post-test discrimination, many people may avoid testing out of fear that the test results could be used against them. While most people will agree that confidentiality of traditional medical information must be respected, genetic information poses particular dilemmas as it can have repercussions for close relatives of individuals who undergo testing. It may affect their right not to know, and interpersonal relationships within the family. Samples collected for newborn screening potentially provide a 'bank' of genetic material, with immense potential value for public health initiatives, epidemiological and laboratory research and commercial products. In India, knowledge of patient rights is almost non-existent. As my empirical research shows, most clients sign consent forms without reading and/or understanding them. Language forms a formidable barrier in this respect. Most consent forms are used primarily to absolve service providers and medical institutions from any liability claims in the future.

The psychological and social impact of genetic testing should not be underestimated. Testing gives rise to anxiety for those waiting to receive results. The safety of tests is an issue, and so is fear of miscarriage. False-negative tests give false reassurances about the ultimate outcome of pregnancy, and false-positive tests lead to unnecessary anxiety and unnecessary abortions. Testing may lead to genetic discrimination by health and life insurance companies and employers, and may have no real benefits for those who lack the means to pay for treatment.

Aggressive marketing of genetic tests raises an additional issue related to the standardisation of the quality of tests and the reliability of test results. Stricter standards for genetic laboratories and standards regarding reliability of interpretation are required. Screening tests should be carried out in accredited, large, centralised laboratories with quality controls. According to one estimate, there are nearly 50,000 clinical laboratories, mostly in urban areas (Kaur 2005). However, only about 40 have obtained accreditation from the National Accreditation Board for Testing and Calibration Laboratories. How to ensure quality assurance standards for laboratories performing genetic tests? This is an extremely relevant question in the Indian context. This concern is voiced by laboratory technicians and geneticists, too (Kaur 2005). The importance of strengthening the public health role in the regulation of genetic tests (improved validity and reliability – 'gold standard') and other genetic services provided primarily by the private sector cannot be emphasised enough.

Finally, an overarching concern is how we can ensure that genetic testing does not widen existing health disparities further, both nationally and internationally (WHO 2002). There is an urgent need for public debates for input into policy settings both for public health spending and applications of genetics in the Indian context. The main priority of the government has to be to reduce inequities in health and health services. 'The citizens have to be *enabled* to take self-responsible decisions' (Dabrock 2006), using the capability and empowerment approach. Health literacy programmes for the public, which include information on genetics and on societal implications (ethical and legal) of developments in the field of human genetics for professionals, need serious attention. Research has shown that decision aids are able to improve the quality and the patient's awareness of prenatal testing decisions; such decision aids should be developed and implemented in the prenatal screening setting. Introducing prenatal screening for congenital defects as part of standard prenatal care should go hand in hand with an adequate system of informing and counselling women about prenatal screening to ensure informed decision-making (Van den Berg et al 2005: 337). Educational materials need to be developed on genetic testing and screening that are culturally sensitive and in an accessible language. Given the linguistic diversity of India, this must include regional languages.

Acknowledgements

This article is based on a chapter presented at the Eighth World Congress of the International Association of Bioethics held in Beijing, 7-9 August 2006.

It is a revised version of an article earlier published in the *Journal for Bioethical Inquiry* (2007) 4: 217-228. The chapter draws on research supported by the Socio-Genetic Marginalisation in Asia Programme (SMAP), funded by The Netherlands Organisation for Scientific Research (NWO) and the International Institute for Asian Studies (IIAS).

I would like to thank Dr I. C. Verma, Head of Genetic Medicine, and his colleagues from the genetics unit and Dr V. K. Khanna, Head of Thalassemia programme at Sir Ganga Ram Hospital, New Delhi, for the cooperation extended to me and allowing me access to their patients. Also, sincere thanks are due to the parents/families of thalassaemic patients who agreed to speak with me.

Notes

1   Public health in this context means activities undertaken by government agencies and financed by taxpayer revenues.
2   1 Indian rupee = US $ 0.02.
3   Discussion paper 'Newborn Screening in India: Current Perspectives' distributed by ICMR and AIIMS, New Delhi, February 2008.

4 Population Genetic Screening for Sickle Cell Anaemia among the Rural and Tribal Communities in India

The Limitations of Socio-ethical Choice

Prasanna Kumar Patra and Margaret Sleeboom-Faulkner

Introduction

This chapter concerns the difficulties related to population genetic screening for sickle cell disease among tribal and rural communities in India. Sickle cell disease is a genetically inherited, commonly encountered haematological disorder that causes high degree of morbidity, mortality and fetal wastage among many Indian tribal and caste communities. Population genetic screening is a public health strategy for detecting future disease risks in individuals or their progeny, for which preventive interventions exist. When this strategy is used as public policy and is applied among marginalised rural and tribal communities, it brings about social and ethical dilemmas regarding healthcare policy choices.

Population-based genetic screening programmes among the rural and tribal communities in India are categorised in the following ways: one, as public health disease prevention programmes aimed at carrier detection; two, as providing genetic counselling to people of childbearing age; and, three, as the offer of alternative treatment options. These intervention attempts have medicalised the issue of genetic screening at the local level, where not only the sickle cell sufferer (homozygous), but sickle cell carrier (heterozygote) individuals, who are otherwise 'normal', and their genetically related kin members, are heaved into the gambit of screening culture.

This chapter problematises the fact that the broad ethical issues such as the principle of autonomy, the requirement of informed consent, the safeguarding of confidentiality, and social issues, such as the empowerment of individuals and communities to exercise choice, are given little weight in publicly mandated genetic screening programmes. Based on primary data collected through cultural anthropological fieldwork among scheduled tribe and caste communities, between March 2006 and May 2007, this chapter focuses on genetic intervention programmes for sickle cell anaemia implemented in rural and tribal areas in India. Here, we contend that, first, the screening programme for sickle cell anaemia in rural and tribal areas in India is based on hapha-zard planning by interventionists, which are both public and private, leading to widespread discrimination and stigmatisation; second, the question of whether to undergo a genetic testing or screening is entirely shaped by the interventionists, where the people or their community have a minor say; and, finally, ill-planned intervention planning that in-cludes population screening brings new forms of inequality.

In various sections of this chapter, we intend to discuss the different rationales put forward by various stakeholders for the genetic screening programmes, the resultant social and ethical issues that emerge from diverse field sites through interventions, and in the concluding section we discuss how comprehensive policy programmes receive public sup-port in comparison to non-comprehensive programmes.

The rationale for population genetic screening of sickle cell anaemia among the rural and tribal communities in India

Advances in the fields of genetics and medical technologies promise great strides in the diagnosis and treatment of many diseases, leading to widespread practices of genetic testing and screening (AAP 2001). Genetic testing and screening are a first step in the State's disease pre-vention and management strategy, which aims to assess the risk of indi-viduals and communities carrying a genetic disease or diseases. It is an established fact that some genetic disorders are more common among certain population groups or communities due to historical and envir-onmental reasons, such as migration patterns, climatic conditions, and occurrences of particular disease-causing viruses or microbes, etc. Sickle cell anaemia is one such genetic disorder, which is unevenly pre-valent throughout the world. With nearly an incidence of 8 in 100,000 people, it is found in almost all populations, but it is most prevalent in people whose ancestors lived in malaria-infested areas (Murray 2002). It affects an estimated 60-70 million people all over the world, and nearly 20 million in India. Out of India's 437 scheduled tribal groups, the heterozygote rate (carrier for the disease) for sickle cell disease ran-ging from 15 per cent to 20 per cent is found among twenty groups, and it is even higher in certain groups (Basu 1994). Sickle cell disease is widespread in tribal as well as non-tribal communities in India, with representative population groups from various regions including: Kondh tribe, Pana and Agaraia castes in eastern India; Bhil, Otkal, Ma-dia, Pawara, and Dhodia tribes from western India and Mullakurumba, Irula, Paiya tribes in southern India who have higher carrier frequencies (TIHF/GAH 2007; Balgir 2005a, b; Kate & Lingojwar 2002). The reporting of these figures, though sporadic and unsystematic, has been done primarily by physical anthropologists and population geneticists who, in the last several decades, have had an academic interest in studying such populations for different reasons at different points in time. In comparison to the scheduled tribes, the prevalence of sickle cell disease is lower among the schedule castes and general caste groups, mainly due to lack of documentation and late interest in these groups by field scientists, apart from other reasons such as the epidemiological link of the disease with high prevalence of malaria in the geographical locations. The genetic intervention programmes, which include community genetic screening, genetic counselling and treatment efforts, mainly focus on communities reported to have a high incidence of sickle cell carriers to prevent further spreading. There exist different intervention strategies and differing rationales amongst different state governments, intervention agencies and the community leaders.

In this chapter we present four different intervention locales that have different natures and strategies in their planning and execution (see Table 4.1). In the state of Chhattisgarh, the intervention programme is focused mainly on a community screening programme based on the strategy of carrying out door-to-door screening for sickle cell anaemia. The Sickle Project is run by the local branch of Indian Red Cross Society, with funding and support from the Chhattisgarh state government. Their approach is to adopt villages in the entire state with a history of reported prevalence for sickle cell anaemia and screen the total population.

The Gujarat state has initiated a comprehensive Sickle Cell Project on a private-public partnership basis, with more focus on screening and counselling. Initially, the project has been implemented in four districts of the state and there are plans to cover the whole state in future. The approach is to screen the population who come to its identified screening centres as referral cases or those who come voluntarily. It also organises regular screening camps in tribal and rural areas of the state. The funding for the intervention in the state comes mainly from the Gujarat state government and partly from the central government.

In the state of Orissa we focused on two locales; Sundargarh and Phulbani districts. Though in both districts there are communities with a high prevalence of sickle cell anaemia (e.g. Kondh tribe and Pana caste in Phulbani and Agaria caste in Sundargarh), there are no intervention strategies or healthcare preparations present at public or private levels. However, there is a Sickle Cell Project run by the Burla Medical College and Hospital at Sambalpur, which organises periodic screening camps at various places in the region, and also provides screening and

Table 4.1 Health intervention programmes at different locales in India

State	Location	Type of communities studied	Structure of intervention effort	Organisations involved	Main objective or strategy	History of intervention
Chhattisgarh	Arang Block of Raipur district	Sahu Teli (schedule caste)	Public-private Partnership	Indian Red Cross Society and Government of Chhattisgarh	Door-to-door population screening	Project started in 2005-06
Gujarat	Valsad	Dhodia tribe	Public-private partnership	Valsad Raktdan Kendra	Screening and counselling	Old programme for over a decade and the new programme for last two years
Orissa	Sundargarh and Phulbani districts	Agaria caste and Kondh tribe	Public at one site and no intervention at other	Burla Medical Hospital (BMC) and Sundargarh and Phulbani District Hospitals	Screening at BMC and no strategies at Phulbani and Sundargarh	At BMC for one year
Maharashtra counselling and treatment	Dhadgaon tahsil of Nandurbar district Programme with different objectives have been ongoing for two decades	Bhil and Pawara tribes	Private (NGO)	Maharashtra Arogya Mandal	Screening	

counselling facilities to patients who visit the hospital and the screening centre within the hospital on the basis of referral.

The intervention programme at Dhadgaon Tahsil in Maharashtra state, another locale, is run by an NGO named Maharashtra Arogya Mandal on a charity basis. It provides mass genetic testing at a nominal price and offers treatment for free. The camp is regularly held every two months, and people voluntarily come to the campsite for carrier screening, health check-ups and free medicine.

Socio-ethical concerns related to screening for sickle cell disease among marginalised communities: The question of choice

Although population screening programmes may help to improve public health in the context of tribal and small-scale communities in India, they are also laden with social and ethical challenges. There are issues related to the traditional or cultural specificity of communities, and issues related to the nature of the disease targeted, e.g. genetic diseases. For instance, information yielded by genetic tests is familial. This means that the study results of one person may have direct health implications for other family and community members who are genetically and socially related. Secondly, in the context of some communities, the psychological, social and financial risks are more profound than the risks from genetic testing and screening. For example, psychosocial risks such as discrimination, social stigma, guilt, anxiety, impaired self-esteem and inability to make social choices can be more challenging than the genetic screening results. Thirdly, the limited predictive capability of genetic screening; for instance, the sickle cell anaemia gene has differential genetic expressions for individuals, making it complicated to diagnose and to prescribe any remedial measure with accuracy. Finally, many genetic conditions, including sickle cell anaemia, have limited or no permanent curative options available to financially marginalised people, rendering the value of genetic screening to those communities questionable. Apart from these commonly encountered socio-ethical concerns, there are other community-specific social and ethical issues meriting attention, which we address in the following sections.

Screening and test results: associated stigma and other ethical issues

In the context of rural and tribal societies, identification of carriers for sickle cell anaemia (heterozygotes) is a crucial addition to identifying the sufferers (homozygous). Though identifying carriers in a population

is a way forward in preventing the disease from spreading, it may stig-
matize some individuals and lead to the undesired medicalisation of life
conditions of the entire community.

At our study locales, such as Dhadgaon in Maharashtra and Valsad in
Gujarat, the screening programmes are based on voluntary participation. People come to the bi-monthly screening camp organised by the
Maharashtra Arogya Mandal at Dhadgaon Tehsil headquarters on a referral basis, or voluntarily, having been influenced by relatives or peer
groups who have already been screened at the camp. At Valsad, people
come to the screening centre based at Valsad Raktdan Kendra, a voluntary healthcare centre offering carrier screening for sickle cell anaemia
for over a decade, on referral or voluntary basis. However, at Arang in
the state of Chhattisgarh, participation to the screening programme is
to some extent obligatory. Even through participation in the intervention
programme is not compulsory for all the villagers, the village committee's direct involvement and its impression that the programme is beneficial to the entire village community has made every individual perceive it as obligatory. At Arang, as part of its intervention strategy, the
local Red Cross Society adopts some villages and *Panchayats*[1] that re-
portedly have higher degrees of sickle cell prevalence rate. It organises
screening camps as part of the free health check-up camp,[2] which the
local people feel obliged to attend. Organisers proclaim that this intervention will help in preventing the spread of the disease from their
community. Hence it became the social duty and responsibility of every
individual in the village to support this mass screening initiative.

From a public health perspective, mass carrier detection programmes
are considered the first step towards a better management of the disease prevention programme. After the carrier status of screened individuals is identified, the target individuals, mainly unmarried adolescents
and people of the childbearing age group, are provided with genetic
counselling in order to take decisions with regard to marriage and issues about having children. However, identification of carriers raises a
number of social and ethical dilemmas, as a significant concern raised
by carrier screening programmes is the possibility for individual and
community to misunderstand the state of being a carrier. Confusion
about the difference between being an asymptomatic carrier for a genetic condition and being affected with the condition may lead to stigma
and discrimination, as well as adverse psychological reactions in those
being screened. Additional disadvantages of knowing one's carrier status include an alteration of self-esteem, a negative impact on family perception of marriage and child, increased anxiety, blaming oneself or parents for the condition and possible discrimination against a child's education.

In the selected study areas, there were different responses to the intervention efforts in regard to carrier identification. In Arang in Chhattisgarh, where the local Red Cross Society, along with the state government, arranged a door-to-door screening programme, the village community leaders voluntarily helped organising the camp in their village, helped the interventionist medical staffs to collect blood samples and do the carrier tests. The first author (PP) interviewed a village committee member, Mr A. Sahu, from Chapridi village in Raipur district (translation by first author):

PP: How did the screening camp happen in your village?

AS: When we came to know from a doctor that our Sahu samaj (Sahu society) is mostly affected by this disease and to prevent the disease from spreading, we needed to know our carrier status. So we asked the Red Cross Society at Raipur to adopt our village and organise the screening. Therefore it was our initiative.

PP: Now, do you think the carrier screening has helped you, I mean the villagers?

AS: I cannot definitely say yes or no. A good thing that happened is that now we know who risks developing the disease. If the person wants to, he or she can take preventive measures. Also the diseased individuals are diagnosed and identified, making it helpful for them to ask for medical help directly, without having to undergo a further test. But the bad thing that we did not foresee when we allowed the screening programme to take place in our village is that now the identified carriers, about 20 per cent of the total village, are being stigmatised. Though the doctors say they are normal, they are depressed and traumatised. Some even have the same symptoms as the sufferers. They are confused and worried about what kind of reproductive decisions they or their children will have to make in future.

PP: When did you receive the test results?

AS: The medical team collected our blood and did the testing here in the camp, in our village. But they gave us the result sheet and the colour cards three days later.

PP: To whom did they give the result sheet and the colour cards?

AS: They gave that to the village committee members (their representative).

PP: Then how did you communicate the results to the carriers and the diseased persons?

AS: We called the diseased persons [23 persons in total] or their family head to the Panachayat office, and gave them the colour cards[3] and the test results. As for the carriers, since there were as many as about 400, we just distributed the cards through our volunteers.

PP: Did anyone have any complaint about the open distribution of his/her test result?

AS: Mm ... not really! By and large there was no problem. But some did not like it. They wanted the result to be confidential, especially the parents of unmarried girls. They were concerned about the repercussions. But most of the diseased individuals have symptoms that are difficult to conceal. One or two people out of the 23 identified diseased were surprised and shocked to learn that they are diseased. They also did not trust the result and suspected its authenticity.

PP: Now it is already more than one year ago that this screening camp was held in your village. How do you look at its positive and negative impacts?

AS: What positive impacts? It is all about false promise. We were promised that all 23 sickle-positive patients would get regular free medical check-ups and blood transfusions from the Red Cross Society at Raipur for 21 years. Forget about 21 years; they did not give it to us even once, when we approached them this year. Rather, our village committee had to spend nearly ten thousand rupees from its fund, which was not reimbursed. Many people are feeling depressed and traumatised for the unnecessary revelations of their health status due to the test, which was unnecessary. The only good thing that came from this is that we know now that this disease is not good for our Samaj's (society) future, and that we need to take steps to prevent it. But we really do not know how and what will be its impact.

This case study reveals many typical issues involved in genetic screening in rural and tribal set-ups. First, there are the issues of risk perception and of making a choice to avoid that risk. Here, the village leadership decided to invite the medical screening team at the Red Cross Society to screen the entire village. It was initiated by the people themselves. Second is the issue of breaching confidentiality. The screening medical team or the interventionist did not show sufficient professional acumen in maintaining a scientific procedure of confidentiality while disclosing the test results to the carriers and affected individuals. In an open society like a rural caste village, where health information of an individual is subjected to public scrutiny, the open distribution of test results made many villagers feel embarrassed and later brought them stigma and discrimination. Female members, especially the unmarried females, were more often the subjects of stigmatisation. Thirdly, there is the issue of false promises made by the interventionists. The villagers felt that they had been let down by the interventionists when they did not deliver what they had promised while collecting the blood sample or doing the screening.

Informing and seeking informed consent

The concept of informed consent, with its emphasis on individual autonomy, personal decision-making and the protection of privacy, has been a central component in research ethics. The idea of informed consent – the requirement to inform participants in a research study of all planned experiments – has accordingly become the gold standard of research ethics (Elger & Caplan 2006; Kegley 2004). The Council of International Organizations of Medical Sciences (CIOMS) guidelines give the most concise definition of informed consent:

> A decision to participate in research made by a competent individual who has received the necessary information, has adequately understood the information, and after considering the information, has arrived at a decision without having been subjected to coercion, undue influence, inducement or intimidation. (CIOMS 2002)

Though the ethical guidelines prepared by the Indian Council of Medical Research (ICMR) and the Department of Biotechnology (DBT) urge researchers to seek informed consent from research subjects, in practice researchers do not. There are many impediments to informed consent at the grass-roots level, especially while conducting screening programmes among rural and tribal communities. Common forms of impediments include illiteracy, poverty, paternalistic attitudes, cultural barriers, implicit forms of coercion, situational pressure, resistance from healthcare professionals and a lack of, or ineffective, regulatory mechanisms (Patra & Sleeboom-Faulkner 2007a).

In the context of universal carrier screening programmes, certain questions need to be asked, such as should screening be conducted without prior consent, considering that it can yield genetic information that some parents would prefer not to know. How should the information about sickle cell traits be conveyed, and to whom? In the absence of trained counsellors in the intervention team, which is usually the case in India, who provides advice? Case studies at various locales in India show that the importance and requirement of informed consent when conducting community-based genetic carrier screening is not duly recognised, either by the interventionists or the individual participants concerned. In other words, the obligatory ethical principles that

ICMR and DBT expect from researchers and interventions are not followed. Some believe that it is not required for the genetic health intervention programme for sickle cell anaemia, where the blood samples are used 'only once' and when the study is only meant to identify carrier status, that is, not for further research, as is the case in biobanking. For instance, Dr Dalla, Director of Sickle Cell Project Chhattisgarh, said:

> Yes, we do understand the need of informed consent, but what is its need in this type of research? We are not collecting bio-samples and keeping it for future research purposes. It is just a one-time collection and moreover we want to help people in some ways. They do not know what is good for them. The moment you start talking about your project and all that stuff that bioethicist argue, they will just run away.

Others believe that the application of informed consent will unnecessarily act as a hindrance to intervention projects, viewing informed consent as merely an administrative exercise. Dr Kate, who has been working for three decades on sickle cell anaemia among the tribal population groups of Maharashtra, and the present Project Head of Sickle Cell Project at Dhadgaon, said:

> Informed consent is a good thing to practice. We do tell people and take their opinion, but it's impractical to practise the way guidelines expect, especially in tribal areas. Here, people do not understand anything. If you ask for their consent or opinion on anything, they will seek your opinion in return and ask you to give them a decision. It will just be an administrative exercise, but nothing more than that, particularly in our kind of intervention projects.

People in policymaking bodies, such as the ICMR, have different views. The ICMR stipulates that the concept of informed consent need to be exercised in all situations and in all kinds of biological research involving humans as research subjects. Dr Nandini Kumar, Deputy Director of ICMR, said:

> Even if the present bioethical guideline prepared by the ICMR is not yet a law, we expect all researchers and institutes to abide by it and follow it in true spirit. Informed consent should ideally be practised and exercised in all types of biological sample collection and research, including population genetic or epidemiological studies.

Community leaders across study locales feel they are not adequately informed about the purpose of screening and what kind of practical expectations they can have from the study. As one villager from Chapridi village in Chhattisgarh said:

> I did not know how this screening will help me. I just came because I heard some doctors will be visiting the camp and they will check us free of cost and give free medicine. I thought the blood test will at least tell me what kind of health problem I have. But, even after one year I do not know what disease I have. And what happened to my blood that they took. No. No. I do not know anything. (translation by first author).

From the above statements by different stakeholders, it is evident that, though informed consent is recognised as an important tool in protecting the rights of the participant, it is discounted due to lack of awareness on the part of participants, and regarded by interventionists as an unnecessary administrative burden.

Issues of gender and inequality

Discrimination based on gender is one of the most salient forms of discrimination as a consequence of the genetic carrier-screening programme for sickle cell anaemia in rural and tribal areas in India. Gender-based genetic discrimination refers to discrimination directed against an individual, based solely on his or her sex in the context of family and society, in cases of an apparent or perceived genetic variation from the 'normal' human genotype. In all four study locales, women are discriminated against on the basis of their genotypic conditions in the sphere of marriage negotiation, family life at their in-laws' house and in economic life. The following are case studies that show how genetic test results have adverse effects on people's lives, especially the women.

Case study 1: How a young woman's marital life became the first casualty of genetic testing

Kanak is a 24-year-old divorced Kondh tribal woman from the Phulbani district of Orissa. She is the eldest of two sisters, living with their father, who have married after their mother died some five years ago. They subsist on farm labour. Kanak is a sickle cell sufferer. Kanak entered a 'love' marriage when she was 15 years old. She used to fall sick at least twice a year, especially during winter and summer seasons. She did not know why. When her mother died in the district hospital after complex health-related complaints, doctors suspected a problem. They advised Kanak and her sister to have a blood test and both of them were positive for sickle cell anaemia. Doctors advised her to bring her husband for a test to ascertain his sickle cell status, but he refused. They advised Kanak not to have children without testing the carrier status of her husband. This bit of information created a furore in her family life. Her husband, after coming to believe that Kanak had an incurable health problem, concluded that she could not produce a healthy child, and divorced her after four years of conflict. Now Kanak says she is leading a miserable life with no money for treatment.

In this case, a young woman was divorced from her husband based on the preliminary test results of her blood sample. As a female, she was blamed and discriminated against.

Case study 2: Dhanti Bai carrying a 'bad' child! A story of suspicion and agony

Dhanti Bai is a 19-year-old Bhil-Pawara tribal woman living in a village near Dhadgaon Tahsil in the Nandurbar district in Maharashtra. She has been married for nine months and is four months pregnant. She has had no severe health-related complaints. However, at the insistence of social health workers in the area, she went to the genetic carrier screening camp to test her carrier status for sickle cell disease, a testing effort organised by the Maharashtra Arogya Mandal at Dhadgaon HQ. She tested positive for sickle cell disease. Although the test result was given to her personally, it somehow became publicly known to other family members and relatives. She was subjected to severe stigma and mental stress. She wanted to know the status of the foetus that she was carrying, but the doctors at the camp advised her to go to Mumbai, the nearest place where a prenatal diagnosis facility is available. To go to Mumbai, approximately 500 kilometres from Dhadgoan Tahsil, she needed a considerable amount of money for travel, in addition to the testing fees. In the meantime, Dhanti Bai's mother-in-law and sister-in-law were blaming Dhanti Bai for carrying a possibly unhealthy child. She was also blamed for the fact that her family had not revealed her true health status when they were negotiating her marriage. Now she is worried about the future health of the child, as she knows that there is variability in the expression of sickle cell genes. Dhanti is cursing her fate, knowing about her disease status when pregnant. She would prefer not to know, especially as she does not have access to suitable medical facilities.

This case study brings many social and ethical questions into picture. First, it raises the question of the desirability of advising someone to take a genetic test when they are not aware of the symptoms of the disease. Second, how do we tackle the issue of confidentiality of test results in a close-knit society, such as a tribal village, where information pertaining to individuals is shared with family members and neighbours in the village? Finally, how do we tackle the issue of prenatal screening in situations where healthcare facilities are neither affordable nor available?

There are individuals who take part in mass genetic screening, considering it as an opportunity to know their health risk and take necessary preventive measures in order to reduce that risk. They take genetic tests voluntarily and influence others to go for them. Kanta from Dhodia tribe is such an example.

Case study 3: Genetic screening as an opportunity to prevent the disease from spreading

Kanta is a 32-year-old woman belonging to the Dhodia tribe in the Valsad district of Gujarat. She is a sickle cell carrier and a mother to three children, one of whom is a sickle cell patient. She came to know about her sickle cell status and also the status of her three children only after she had given birth to all of them. She does not want to have any more children because she is now aware of the fact that her husband is also a carrier, which can cause a child to inherit the disease. She said that when she heard from another woman in the village about this disease, she immediately thought that her second child might be a sufferer. She took him to the screening centre for a carrier test and he was found to be a sickle positive patient. Then she persuaded her husband to take the test and also took the test for the other two children. Her husband is a carrier and the two other children are normal. She thinks that since women have to bear most of the burden of taking care of the diseased child, she should take a more active role in taking the test and in deciding whether or not to have another child. She now wants to create awareness in her village among the people about the disease and persuade people to take the test, so that they can take preventive as well as lifestyle-related curative measures to reduce the disease burden of their family as well as that of the community.

Avoidance of risk is one of the main motives for people to take part in genetic screening programmes. Some also influence others to undergo screening, so that they may be able to take preventive measures. In this process, other family and kin members are pulled into the gambit of screening. Peer or relative pressure makes asymptomatic or otherwise 'normal' individuals participate in screening activities, leading to the spread of screening culture.

The therapeutic gap and unmet needs

It has proved far easier for scientists to develop tests for genetic diseases than to devise effective intervention methods to prevent manifestations in people who are born affected (Holtzman & Shapiro 1998). This so-called therapeutic gap for sickle cell disease has been a big problem in both developed and developing countries, and the gap further widens when it comes to marginalised communities living in developing countries. Treatment for sickle cell anaemia is usually aimed at avoiding crises, relieving symptoms and preventing complications. If one has sickle cell anaemia, he or she will need to have regular check-ups for her or his red blood cell count and monitor it. There may also be a requirement for treatment from specialists at a hospital or sickle cell anaemia clinic. Treatment may include medication to reduce pain and prevent complications, blood transfusions and supplemental oxygen, as well as bone marrow transplants. Bone marrow transplantation offers the only potential cure for sickle cell anaemia (Charache et al 1995). The facilities are expensive and the technology is unavailable to people living in developing countries. Whenever and wherever it is available, very few people find a suitable donor for transplantation.

Patients with sickle cell disease require continuous treatment, even when they do not have a painful crisis. Supplementation with folic acid, an essential element in producing red blood cells, is required because of the rapid red blood cell turnover. The purpose of treatment is to manage and control symptoms, and to try to limit the frequency of crises. Hydroxyurea is the first drug approved for the causative treatment of sickle cell anaemia, and was shown to decrease the number and severity of attacks and also shown to possibly increase the survival time of those affected (Charache et al 1995; Steinberg et al 2003). However, many affected people in developing countries cannot afford to buy this medicine. Other new medicines such as butyric acid, clotrimazole and nitric oxide, and treatment efforts such as bone marrow transplantation and gene therapy, which are prescribed or available in developed countries, are not available to the patients of marginalised communities living in a developing country such as India.

The kind of treatment facilities that are available to people in our study areas are common pain relievers, such as analgesics, and some suggestions as part of counselling on how to take some lifestyle-related precautions. In one study site, at Dhadgaon Tahsil in Maharashtra state in the Maharashtra Arogya Mandal (MAM), an NGO is providing some

Ayurvedic herbal medicine which it claims will increase the red blood cell count in the body. It provides the medicine to the sufferers free of charge. However, the Ayurvedic medicine is neither approved by the drug controlling authority of India, nor are the NGO doctors sure about its efficacy. Dr Shirode, a member of the medical team that works at the MAM's screening camp, said:

> We are not quite sure about the drug's efficacy and whether it really helps to increase the red blood cells. Our assessment is based on the common observation that people are feeling good and think that their health condition has improved. And that should be OK. It is based on traditional Ayurvedic medicine systems. It has no side effects. One good thing about this free medicine distribution is that it gives immense psychological and moral support to the patient taking medicine. You know, for these poor people hydroxyurea is not affordable; they have no other source. So this is a great help, even we are not very sure of its exact efficacy. (translation by first author).

Many married couples, of whom both are sickle cell carriers, are shattered when told to avoid having children. Even though both of them are 'normal', that is, asymptomatic, they worry about the genetic status of their offspring. The counsellor tells them about the possibility of prenatal diagnosis, which can detect the defective genetic condition of the foetus. In most of the tribal and rural areas, modern facilities for prenatal diagnosis are not available and, even when present, are unaffordable. As one Dhodia tribal woman from Valsad said:

> Now, it is frustrating to know that I am pregnant and that I may be carrying a child that has increased chance of becoming a defective child. There are medical testing facilities available for finding out if the foetus has a problem. But we have to travel to Mumbai for that for which we have no money. We are poor; we cannot afford it. (translation by first author).

There are also cases where people want to access the technology and they have financial resources for doing so, but there is no technology available to them at affordable price and reasonable accessibility in local areas. As one Agaria caste man said:

> I wanted to test my children for the disease after I read in the newspaper that our Samaj is more prone to sickle cell disease than others. But there is no testing facility nearby. The local government should establish a testing facility at least at the district

hospital. If I have to take the test, now I have to travel to another district, which is very far away and I have to spend a lot of money for a simple test. Why is the government not sensitive and considerate enough to make this available to us? (translation by first author).

As we have witnessed in the above cases, there exists a gap between the needs of people affected by sickle cell anaemia and therapeutics available in the field. Again, the gap is widened in the context of marginalised communities, where the healthcare infrastructural facilities are poorly managed. The therapeutic gap is a complex issue of medical technological developments in the field and distributional aspects of such technologies available locally. Developing countries, especially marginalised communities living therein, suffer from these dual limitations. An intervention programme needs to be comprehensive in taking into account the needs of the people. For instance, a screening programme needs to be followed by basic treatment facilities available locally, provision of counselling to the targeted individuals and wider awareness generation in the community.

Cultural and social tradition

Genetic carrier screening at community level is marred by two contrasting claims and responses. Public health experts and population genetic interventionists are concerned about improving the overall health of a community, by preventing deleterious or defective genes from entering the gene pool, through technological and policy interventions. Their major concern is to encourage the birth of healthy children and avoid the birth of children that they consider as a burden on parents, families and the state. Those who oppose such interventions on social and cultural grounds maintain that the natural process of biosocial forces in a society should not be tampered with. They believe in maintaining the 'purity' of the groups' biological as well as cultural practices.

For certain communities 'group purity' and tradition have immense value, which they try to preserve at any cost, even at the cost of perceptible risk to their lives. The case study among the Bhil tribes from Dhadgaon in Maharashtra shows that the Bhils did not participate in the community carrier screening programme for the sickle cell anaemia when it was initiated by the Maharashtra Arogya Mandal (MAM) some two decades ago. Their non-cooperation with the intervention effort was due to the cultural factor of 'purity', believing that they belong to the powerful warrior *Rajput* clan, whose blood is all-pure and powerful – so there is no possibility of any defect in their blood for which they might need to take a genetic test. As Dr Shirode puts it:

> In the beginning it was difficult for us to get local people's support for the screening camp, as people refused to take part on cultural ground. Bhils then believed that sickle cell disease is a problem that lies in the 'blood' and, since they belong to a powerful warrior class, their blood is 'superior' and 'pure'. They believed that we, the project staffs, are trying to dilute their group purity. We had to work hard to perusade them. It took a long time and even today, many Bhil believe in those lines. (translation by first author).

The community-based genetic carrier screening programmes have a most visible impact on marriage. Marriage has both biological and social significance for a community, in carrying forward a particular set of genetic profiles from generation to generation through mating in a biological sense, to maintaining social bonds through relations. For prevention of genetically-based public health problems, such as sickle cell anaemia, regulation of mating in its biological sense and marriage in its social sense is crucial. Medical doctors and genetic counsellors involved in intervention programmes support the regulation of marriage (mate selection): a process whereby a carrier should avoid marrying another carrier or sufferer to avoid the expansion of deleterious genes in the population. As part of an awareness programme, intervention teams publish and distribute leaflets and pamphlets, explaining pictographically different sets of permutation and combinations of genotypic characters. The materials indicate how particular types of mating should be avoided. Interventionists popularise a slogan as part of their awareness programme by urging people to match the 'genetic *kundli*' in place of traditional horoscope '*janma kundali*'.[4]

Some community leaders are critical about this strategy adopted by the interventionist in the field study areas. Mr A. Sahu, President of *Sahu Samaj*, an association of Sahu caste people in Raipur of Chhattisgarh, said:

> This sickle cell screening programme is a dangerous thing for our Sahu samaj. They are just exaggerating the health risk to the Sahu community. I think there is a motive behind this to malign our caste and to dilute our culture. If this risk is as high as they are saying, then our community should have vanished long before or we would have a higher rate of diseased people. They want us to change our marriage pattern, to avoid us getting married among our caste groups. They even advise people not to get

married or not to have children. This is against our Samaj and we will oppose this. Please, tell me who is not at risk: who is free from disease? Why should I abandon my dreams and happiness for something which has no cure and which cannot be diagnosed properly with certainty? (translation by first author).

The situation is different at another study locale. The community leaders of Agaria caste group from Sundargarh in Orissa generally approve the risk perceptions and disease prevention strategy that are put forward by the medical doctors and interventionists. As Mr Prabodh Patel, an advocate and young Agaria leader from the area, said:

We need to be pragmatic. There are reports that show that we Agarias have one of the highest incidence rates for sickle cell disease. In all our Gudis [caste associations] and annual functions we urge to our fellow members to voluntarily do the sickling test to avoid marriage between two carriers. Ours is a small community with a population of a few thousand, so it is difficult to find a suitable life partner. This carrier-based mate selection will add to our problem. We did not encourage anybody marrying outside our caste, but looking at the risk to our society from this disease, we may have to adopt a strategy where intercaste marriage should be possible. I know it is going to be difficult to convince my fellow caste-men, but we will have to do this. (translation by first author).

We find differences in perception about the screening intervention across study sites and communities, depending on the kind of intervention strategy, cultural background of the community and socio-economic conditions. For instance, in study sites such as Dhadgaon in Maharashtra and Valsad in Gujarat, where screening is followed by treatment efforts and counselling, respectively, there is relatively better support for the intervention programme, in comparison to study sites at Arang block in Chhattisgarh, where there was only a random screening intervention without follow-up counselling or treatment effort. Similarly, the Agaria caste groups have a positive view, and they support the screening, in contrast to Sahu caste communities from Chhattisgarh. The Agarias, being educationally and economically better off than the Sahus, are more open and less conservative in their attitude towards the intervention and voluntarily attempt to regulate their social marriage system.

Challenges in counselling

As genetic health intervention programmes are based on the premise of risk, genetic counselling as part of the intervention strategy plays a growing role in the evaluation and risk estimation of individuals and families with suspected genetic conditions. Genetic counselling ideally is an interactive education and communication process, whose purpose is to evaluate an individual's or group's potential risk of developing a specific type of genetic disease. The ultimate goal of the education and communication process is to help the individual and other family members make informed and appropriate decisions about genetic testing options and preventive strategies (Kate 2000; Raz & Atar 2004). When this ideal counselling framework is applied in the field situation, especially in conditions where the counsellor's confrontation is not limited to a subject individual or to his or her immediate family or kin members, but rather to a larger social or community network, it represents a new direction in community genetic health intervention and raises some particularly interesting and difficult issues.

The common problems encountered in the field in regard to counselling are: (1) the little attention that counselling has received from interventionists, even though the on-the-ground reality demands a greater role for counselling; (2) the lack or shortage of trained genetic counsellors adds to the existing levels of stigma and discrimination as a side-effect of insensitive or faulty counselling; and (3) genetic counsellors, wherever located, are overburdened with other expected professional duties and sandwiched between moral positions and practical situational demands.

Of the four locales we have studied, only at two places, at Raipur in Chhattisgarh and Valsad in Gujarat, are there genetic counsellors available, even though they are few in number and are not professionally trained as genetic counsellors. At two other places, in Dhadgaon in Maharashtra and Phulbani in Orissa, there are no such counsellors. The reasons that are cited are lack of funds to recruit counsellors, and lack of appreciation for their role in the intervention effort, as it is commonly believed that medical doctors or other paramedical staff who are regular members of the intervention group can handle the job of counsellor. The case study from Dhadgaon Sickle Project camp reveals this fact. There is a Sickle Cell Camp every two months that is held for two days by a charitable trust called the Maharashtra Arogya Mandal, at Dhadgaon district headquarters in the Maharashtra state. Around 400 old and new patients visit this camp, where services such as blood testing, health check-ups and free medicines for pain are provided with a 'nominal' service charge of twenty Indian rupees per test. There is no genetic counsellor appointed. The medical doctors and supporting staff provide basic information and attend to patients if they have any queries. However, considering the high number of patients (around 400 in two days) and staff (five or six medical and support staff), it is not possible for them to attend to the needs of the people. Dr S. L. Kate, who is in charge of the Sickle Project, said of the issue of genetic counselling:

> We are working in this area for several decades and our main objective is to screen as many people as possible and provide them some kind of treatment. We know the importance of counselling, which is very much necessary. But for that you need two things: one, money to recruit a trained counsellor which is difficult as ours is a charitable trust and we do not have sufficient fund for that; the second point is getting a counsellor who is from this local area, who understands the local language and culture. Otherwise it will be a mess.

Although there is a growing recognition that genetic counselling needs to be an inseparable part of community-based genetic intervention strategy, lack of funding in appointing genetic counsellors and the lack of trained genetic counsellors to take up the post in intervention sites are cited as the main challenges.

Even though India shoulders one-third of the global burden of genetic diseases (Balgir 2001; Verma & Bijarnia 2002), there are no specialised institutes to train genetic counsellors who can work in diverse field situations where there is a need for them. In the real situation, the people who end up doing jobs as genetic counsellors are drawn from various academic backgrounds with minimal exposure to the issues that they are expected to deal with. The work of a counsellor is a tricky job, especially in the context of community carrier screening programmes where the genetic and social linkages between target individuals, their family members, and the community are 'open' and 'accessible'. In a typical case, an identified sickle cell carrier is counselled to take on responsibility on behalf of the family and kin members, and is advised to bring whomever he or she thinks at risk of being another carrier or sufferer to the screening facility in order to help the counsellor map the risk falling on the individual and family members. Any kind of misjudgement and misguidance on the part of the counsellor may bring stigma and discrimination to communities, especially tribal and small communities, which follow local cultural and traditional norms and values that may not be attuned with scientific practices in counselling. For example, if after being identified as a carrier for sickle cell anaemia, a married woman is advised by a counsellor to bring her husband to the testing centre, this may create problem for her. She is usually blamed for the disease and is made responsible for carrying the 'problem'. In other cases, individuals who take the initiative to inform other kin members to take genetic testing are blamed for medicalising them and bringing 'unnecessary' trauma and stigma to their lives.

The job of a genetic counsellor, dealing with management of risk that is interwoven with individuals with family relations and within small communities, is particularly difficult. In our study areas, we encountered genetic counsellors who are dealing with multiple professional tasks, as medical doctors or paramedical staff, with counselling as an additional duty. They are overburdened with their work, and have little time to understand the broad-based information and cultural factors in order to provide adequate counselling to needy individuals or families. The number of people who seek counselling is large, considering the number of counsellors at work at any one centre. Another difficulty that the counsellors face is the dilemma of adhering to professional moral positions or practical situational demands. As counsellors, they are supposed to avoid giving directive counselling or being paternalistic. However, in practical field situations, where impoverished subjects rely too much on the counsellor to take decisions on issues that they are not sure of, due to the complexity of the issues and their inaptitude to comprehend the consequences, it adds additional pressure for the counsellors to be objective and neutral. As Dr Varsha, who is a homeopathic medical doctor and works as a counsellor at the Valsad Raktdan Kendra in Gujarat, said: 'I become very personal and give so many suggestions and guidance to patients and sometimes I am forced to take decisions for people on their behalf. I then doubt my job, if I am working as a counsellor or as a social worker!' This illustrates the situational confusions that the medical doctors and counsellors experience at the grassroots level.

The issue of choice

The subject of genetic health intervention is a complex issue of choice. It starts from the issue of conceiving sickle cell anaemia as a health risk for certain individuals and their communities, and devising policy programmes to intervene in order to prevent the disease from affecting future generations. At various places and occasions, the decision to take part in mass screening programmes is not adequately backed by informed choice, and decision-making by individuals or communities puts a question mark on the paternalistic attitude of the interventionist or the state machinery. The importance of informed consent is not recognised by either the participants or the intervening authorities, and needs to be strengthened after giving proper consideration to the common impediments identified, and also in taking necessary steps in creating conditions that uphold the true spirit of the concept of informed consent. Another problem area is the way communities are selected for a particular kind of intervention, and the scientific explanations provided in selecting them for intervention. Furthermore, whether people from a community have any voice in the whole process of decision-making for intervention needs to be examined.

Choices are always prestructured by a range of factors, including limited information and understanding, cultural values and beliefs, family attitudes and influences, faith and religion, and social and economic conditions. 'Informed choice' and 'informed decision-making' in the context of screening programmes is a critical issue to target individuals, and some authors argue that their communities need to be empowered and be provided with informed options by intervening authorities in order to make decisions about matters important to their lives (Gupta 2007).

In the context of this study, a wide gap was observed between the people who are subjects of the screening programme and the people who represent intervention systems or the state, in terms of ability to decide or choose matters related to their healthcare decisions. The former includes diseased individuals, asymptomatic carrier individuals and community leaders, whereas the latter is represented by medical doctors, screening programme coordinators and state health officials who devise the intervention programmes. Even though there are more than twenty tribal communities with a high incidence of sickle cell anaemia with a greater than 20 per cent carrier prevalence rate, only few communities are selected for intervention programmes by the central or state governments, in an arbitrary manner. The genetic intervention approaches have been very different at various locales; for example, in Gujarat the intervention strategy is more extensive and includes screening, counselling and treatment efforts, whereas in Maharashtra it only includes screening and treatment efforts; in Chhattisgarh it only includes screening, albeit relatively systematic, while in Orissa screening takes place quite randomly. Here, the issue returns of the problems associated with different kinds of intervention strategies operating in different locales. Why are there no standardised and comprehensive policy programmes of intervention? And, why is screening not followed by counselling and treatment plans in all locales? More importantly, how are people's choices affected and framed in the different locales?

There is a perceptible tension concerning what kinds of choices people at local level can have about participating in screening programmes. Where screening is made mandatory in a village or a local area with an assertion by the state or the interventionist that it is the best public health prevention programme available to them, individuals have little

leeway. At the same time, even if the programme is of a coercive nature, the view exists among many people that it is an opportunity for
them to get healthcare facilities otherwise not available to them. Absence or non-availability of basic healthcare facilities at local levels in tribal and rural areas in regard to the detection of and cure for sickle cell
disease is a limiting factor in people's decision whether to participate in
the mandatory screening programme or not, because it is the *only*
meaningful healthcare they can access. As Arati Sahu, a middle-aged
woman from Chapridi village in Chhattisgarh, who has one sufferer
and one carrier child, said:

> I took my children to the camp [for sickle cell screening] for the
> test, because we were told that doctors and nurses would be
> there, and that the health check-up and medicine would be free.
> My children used to have some health problems that could not
> be diagnosed at the primary hospital, so I thought it would be a
> good opportunity for us. Also, our village committee members
> asked us to visit the camp without fail. So, not going there would
> have been a bad thing. (translation by first author).

For some people, the ability of genetic screening programmes to 'predict' the development of sickle cell anaemia is a dilemma. On the one
hand, it brings hope for them in knowing their risk and provides a
chance for them to take preventive measures to minimise the risk. On
the other hand, the knowledge of being at risk carries stigma and discrimination. Parents of unmarried girls are the main subjects, and find it
impossible to take a decision. As Mr. Jivan Sahu, a village committee
leader from Chapridi village, said:

> I very much want to know the carrier status of my daughter so
> that we can avoid her marrying another carrier and avoid having
> a sick child, who would be a constant cause of agony to her. But
> if the test result is positive, we will face difficulties in finding a
> suitable boy for her. So it is better not to test her. But it is diffi-
> cult to decide either this or that; it is a really difficult situation.
> (translation by first author).

Choice is about having alternatives to choose from. If one has the
means to use a screening programme as an advantageous opportunity
to understand the risk involved and use that information for his or her
benefit, that can be termed as 'good risk'. Similarly, a lack of means to
make such information advantageous can be seen as a 'bad risk'. Likewise, having access to, or lack of access to, alternatives can make the selection of options a matter of experiencing 'good' or 'bad' choice. Inter-

vention locales (see Table 4.1) with varying strategies provide differing levels and types of alternatives to individuals, making them able or unable to exercise choice. For example, locales where the screening programme is followed by counselling (e.g. Valsad in Gujarat) provide better options to subject individuals to take life decisions than locales where only screening programmes are available (e.g. Raipur in Chhattisgarh). From this point of view, the way in which people's choices are framed can be said to be 'good' or 'bad' experiences.

Concluding remarks

Genetic screening or intervention programmes for sickle cell anaemia in rural and tribal communities in India bring complex and conflicting scenarios into the picture. Public health experts view it as an affirmative action, leading to the prevention of risk in the lives of individuals and their communities. Critics view it as an intrusion in the lives of individuals who are asymptomatic for the disease and who do not wish to be tested. Such people are nevertheless obliged to or pressurised into participation due to the increasing medicalisation of the issue and severe pressure from peers or relatives. For them, this means a limitation in exercising their choice about matters important to them in their lives. The limitations are both intrinsic and extrinsic in nature. Limitations can be found as a result of lack of infrastructure available in the locality, in terms of education, healthcare delivery systems or lack of public awareness about the problem, or it can dwell in the cultural practices of a particular community.

In this chapter, different study locales displayed differing views about the utility of intervention, depending on the kind of intervention strategy applied, the level of their awareness, and the cultural and social matrix of the community. People are usually supportive of the intervention programme when it is comprehensive in nature, for instance, when it includes genetic screening followed by counselling and treatment efforts, as was the case in Dhadgaon in Maharashtra and Valsad in Gujarat. Compared with non-comprehensive strategies witnessed at other study sites, such as in Arang in Chhatishgarh, where one-time mass screening was done without any follow-up, the choices made were experienced as relatively 'good'.

The haphazard nature of screening programmes for sickle cell disease has brought a negative image to screening, especially in some locales where 'bad' choice characterised the intervention. There is a clear need for a more comprehensive healthcare policy programme that facilitates the healthcare needs of sickle cell disease areas according to their culture and socio-economic situation. While formulating these policies, it should take into account the prevalence of disease in communities or areas, the socio-cultural dimensions of the targeted community and the long-term impact of the programme. Individuals and communities need to be empowered to exercise their 'good' choice about health and life for themselves. The interventionist and the state could play a positive role as facilitators but not as decision-makers.

Notes

1   Panchayat may roughly be translated as local level politico-administrative divisions. It includes one or more villages whose population is at least around 5000.
2   Free health check-up camps are special camps organised mainly by voluntary organisations in rural or tribal areas for different purposes. One of the main attractions of such camps is to provide free medical check-ups and distribution of medicine without any charge or minimal charge.
3   At intervention locales such as Dhadgaon in Maharashtra and Chapridi in Chhattisgarh, interventionists distribute 'colour cards' to carriers and sufferers of the disease based on their screening results. A card which is 'full yellow' signifies a sufferer (genotypically homozygous) and the card with half-yellow and half-white signifies a carrier (genotypically heterozygous). The interventionists believe that the distribution of colour cards help in identifying the holder of the card during next medical check-ups and diagnosis. The other purpose is to help common people understand the carrier status and take appropriate action during marital matchmaking.
4   Many communities in India, especially Hindus and some tribal communities, follow matching of horoscopes while choosing a would-be bride or bridegroom as part of their marriage negotiation. For a perfect match, the horoscopes of both the would-be bride and groom need to be matched. The horoscope is based on traditional Hindu mythological moon signs. Now genetic counsellors and interventionists ask people to match their genotypic characters based on genetic tests in place of *janma kundali* (birth horoscope).

5   Predictive Genetic Testing in India

*Renu Saxena, Swati Sharma, Risha Nahar,
Sudha Kohli, Ratna Puri and Ishwar C. Verma*

Introduction

For centuries, people in India have had their hands and horoscopes inspected for a peek into their future. However, use of predictive genetic testing is of recent origin. Formal studies on the subject are few, but our experience of providing genetic counselling to several thousand families with diverse genetic disorders, and a few hundred with adult-onset genetic disorders (Verma et al 2003), has given us an insight into the ethical and social issues related to predictive testing in a multiethnic and multicultural country such as India.

Most of the conflicts that arise from predictive testing in developing countries are similar to those in the West, but some issues are unique. Therefore, the established international guidelines for predictive testing would require some modifications before they could be applied in developing countries.

Predictive genetic testing in practice

Predictive genetic testing in practice can be of many types, which include testing treatable genetic disorders in the early asymptomatic phase (e.g. Wilson's disease); predictive prenatal testing for genetic disorders such as thalassaemia, Duchenne muscular dystrophy (DMD); predictive testing in hereditary cancer syndromes such as adenomatous polyposis coli (APC) and predictive testing in complex multifactorial disorders such as diabetes mellitus (DM), schizophrenia and vitiligo; and Mendelian monogenic disorders of adult onset such as Huntington's disease (HD). These are discussed below.

Testing treatable genetic disorders in the early asymptomatic phase

Predictive genetic testing can be usefully carried out for disorders that are treatable but have an asymptomatic phase. For example, in Wilson's disease, manifestations appear after a few years (over five years of age). In families with an affected child, the siblings can be tested and, if they are found to carry mutations in both alleles, zinc therapy can be initiated, entirely preventing symptoms of the disease. We have done such testing in ten families. Hardly any ethical issues are raised in performing this type of predictive test for the individuals concerned, apart from obtaining the necessary consent, as a positive test result makes possible the prevention of the disease. In such situations, testing in children is also permissible, as treatment can be given before the appearance of symptoms, and the disease manifestations can be totally prevented.

Predictive prenatal testing

Predictive testing during pregnancy for severe disorders is common practice around the world. In India, predictive prenatal testing for disorders such as thalassaemia, Duchenne muscular dystrophy, spinal muscle dystrophy, cystic fibrosis and other genetic disorders is now commonly used in hospitals, as well as testing for the diagnosis of birth defects due to environmental causes. In India, abortion of an affected foetus is permitted up to twenty weeks of gestation. It is significant that even countries with a predominantly Muslim population, such as Pakistan and Iran, have permitted prenatal diagnosis and abortion up to 120 days of gestation in disorders with severe morbidity. The reason for this is not hard to find. The socio-economic cost of looking after a child affected with thalassaemia major is enormous.

The Indian government and insurance companies do not cover the cost of treating children with genetic disorders, except making available subsidised healthcare in the government hospitals. Therefore, the demand for predictive prenatal diagnosis is great. For example, it has comprised 40 per cent of the work in genetic counselling at our centre over the past several years. The figure has risen to 60 per cent during the past year, as biochemical screening of pregnancy for Down's syndrome and neural tube defects (NTD) has become popular. Though ethical dilemmas may exist, prenatal testing does not prompt most people visiting the hospital to discuss the ethical dilemmas of abortion with the doctor. The detection of an abnormal genotype, e.g. Down's syndrome or homozygous beta thalassaemia, is associated in a foetus with a near certainty that the child will suffer from the disease. That is, if the people request a test to prevent the birth of an unhealthy child, the family has already decided to abort any 'abnormal' foetus.

In India, there is the significant issue of determining the gender of the foetus for social reasons, followed by abortion of healthy female foetuses. As this practice became widespread, the government of India passed national legislation forbidding the use of prenatal diagnostic tests and ultrasound for the determination of gender for social reasons, and disclosure of the same to the patient. However, prenatal diagnosis is allowed for legitimate genetic reasons. The penalties for determining fetal gender for social reasons are very stiff in India, and this has led to a significant reduction in abortion of female foetuses. We receive a number of requests for prenatal paternity testing, but as we consider it unethical, we do not perform the prenatal test for this purpose.

Predictive testing in hereditary cancer syndromes

Predictive testing in hereditary cancers is a well-recognised indication around the world. We have also carried this out in a number of instances in India. In developing countries, a major ethical issue in this type of testing is the cost of the test and their non-availability for poor patients. This has limited the uptake of predictive tests in hereditary cancers. The lack of diagnostic facilities for predictive testing in cancer is also a limitation. Predictive testing in familial cancer syndromes is worthwhile, as a positive test allows for a more strict surveillance programme for the early diagnosis of cancer, while a negative test means that the subject need not undergo frequent testing for recognition of cancer.

In India, one question the symptomatic individuals often ask before deciding to go for the test is whether the genetic tests would alter the management of their disease. In one family with adenomatous polyposis coli (APC), the affected father came all the way from Gujarat to Delhi for the genetic test. When he learnt that the test result would not alter his treatment, he went back without getting the test done. The benefit that would accrue to the other family members and to his children was explained to him, but this did not convince him to undergo genetic testing. As his disease became worse and he realised that his end was near, he agreed to get tested, as the knowledge of the mutation would allow his children to be tested to identify whether they would be at risk of developing the same cancer. After identifying the mutation in the APC gene in the father, we tested both children and found them to be normal. This persuaded the affected sister also to go for the test and also to get her daughter tested, although initially she had stoutly resisted any predictive testing. Fortunately, her daughter also tested negative for the mutation.

In another family, the father and two children had hereditary non-polyposis colon cancer. The 55-year-old son was counselled about predictive testing in his children. He said he understood the advantages of testing their children, who were 25 and 20 years old. He then requested us to convince his wife to agree with testing the children. The wife's immediate question was: 'How would this knowledge affect the prospects of their marriage?' In India, the majority of marriages are still ar-ranged. If the sons tested negative that would be fine. However, she felt unable to cope with the eventuality that any of them might test positive for the mutation. Should they tell the prospective partner that their son has the mutation, and a greater likelihood of developing colon cancer? This was the dilemma she could not resolve. Telling the truth would certainly mean the marriage would not take place. She preferred not knowing whether the sons carried the mutation. This would also avoid the conflict of whether to tell or not to tell the prospective partner about it. Predictive testing in such situations raises serious personal and fa-mily dilemmas, for which there are no clear-cut answers.

Predictive testing in complex / multi-factorial disorders

We often receive requests for predictive testing for complex disorders, such as diabetes mellitus (DM), schizophrenia and vitiligo. One or both partners with the disease are generally concerned that their children should not suffer from the disease that has ravaged their lives. One can understand the anxiety of the parents to ask for predictive testing; how-ever, in the current state of knowledge, accurate prediction of these dis-orders is not possible because, in spite of many studies, the currently identified genes confer a relative risk of only about 2.0. Also, there is a large environmental component, which is difficult to characterise. In the present uncertainty, it has been our policy not to offer predictive test for complex disorders such as diabetes or vitiligo.

The situation keeps changing as new information becomes available. For example, the variations in the *TCF7L2* (transcription factor 7-like 2) gene confer a greater risk of diabetes mellitus type 2 than the gene var-iants previously identified. Recognition of such a variation in an indivi-dual is theoretically expected to motivate him/her to make lifestyle changes in diet and physical exercise routine that would reduce the risk of diabetes mellitus. However, it remains to be seen whether possession of such knowledge does lead to a change in lifestyle for that individual. Unless such information becomes available, it would not be entirely right to claim that this fact will lead to a presymptomatic test, and hence to disease prevention (Janssens 2006). Although we have the capability to perform a genetic test, perhaps we should not assume that offering the test is the right course of action. It is important to demon-strate an improvement in total health outcome before offering predic-tive testing in complex disorders.

Mendelian disorders of adult onset

Several ethical issues occur in predictive testing for monogenic disorders with adult onset, but which do not have any specific treatment at present. Huntington's disease is the classic example for this type of predictive genetic testing. In our series of 107 families where a diagnosis of Huntington's disease was made, members of 31 families opted for predictive testing. Three high-risk families chose to go in for prenatal diagnosis. The younger generations, once they learn that one of their parents has an adult-onset disorder, opt for testing of the disorder during their pregnancy, as there is a great desire to avoid the recurrence of the disorder in future offspring, with its associated problems and tensions. In one of the families that underwent prenatal diagnosis, the high-risk parent, whose father suffered from Huntington's disease, was reluctant to get himself tested as he felt unable to cope with the prospect of having the mutation and the likelihood of suffering from the disease in future. For the sake of his foetus, he requested prenatal diagnosis in his wife's pregnancy and did not want to know his status.

We diagnosed spinocerebellar ataxia in 60 families, 2 with SCA1, 34 with SCA2, 4 with SCA3, 1 with SCA6 and 19 with SCA12. The demand for presymptomatic diagnosis was fairly low, as only two families with SCA2 and one family with SCA12 opted for predictive testing. Only one family with SCA2 underwent prenatal diagnosis.

Predictive genetic testing of children for late-onset autosomal dominant disorders such as HD involves many ethical issues. In the West, there is a general consensus not to do predictive testing in children for disorders that have no treatment in the presymptomatic phase. It is considered advisable to let the children take an independent decision regarding testing once they are older. In India, often the parents desire predictive genetic tests of their children, with the ostensible reason that they can plan their lives accordingly. One father, who was a physician, had spinocerebellar ataxia type 12, and wanted his 20-year-old son and 18-year-old daughter to be tested, as this would help him to choose the type of profession they should pursue. He lived in another city and we had no opportunity to personally interview the children. We therefore acceded to the request of the father. Similarly, a father whose wife suffered from Huntington's disease wished to get his three children aged 10 and under tested. This test was refused, as it would have led to discrimination in love, care and upbringing between children who tested normal and those who tested positive.

Characteristics of parties involved

Predictive genetic testing involves interaction of three parties: (1) the counselee, (2) the counsellor, and (3) the genetic laboratory. The characteristics of these three groups, as they exist in India, are discussed below.

The patient or the counselee

Most counselees know that their family members have suffered from the disorder in question, and live under the fear that they may also be afflicted. The development of any symptoms sets alarm bells ringing. They gladly accept testing, if available, to resolve this uncertainty and to know for sure if they have the disease or not.

Most Indians have great faith in God, and many therefore leave it to God, and are prepared to wait and see what the future holds for them, rather than getting tested. However, if treatment were available they would be very willing to get tested in the asymptomatic stage (predictive testing). However, in the current scenario, when there is no treatment available, only some get tested. The reasons for testing vary with the individual, but mostly they wish to have information about their status so that they can plan their own lives, or the lives of their children. Most of the serious dilemmas in predictive testing arise from the fact of non-availability of any treatment that would alter the course of the illness.

Most counselling and genetic testing services in India do not pay much attention to follow-up of patients during the pre-test and post-test stages. This is mainly due to lack of trained genetic counsellors in India. Patients, especially those with negative test results, are not given much attention; however, some studies have revealed that such individuals can have unpredictable post-test reactions and need to be counselled with frequent follow-ups.

An important issue is the comparative lack of scientific knowledge among the many patients who come from lower socio-economic strata, or from the rural areas. Explaining to them the science behind predictive tests is a challenging task. It becomes imperative to ensure (by indirect means) that they have understood what is being explained to them. It is often necessary to repeat the counselling. A written letter given at the end of the counselling or later would be useful, but in light of the doctors' busy schedule, and the lack of secretarial services, this is often not possible.

Economic indicators for India are revealing. In 2005, The Gross National Income per capita was US $ 720, the total adult literacy rate was 61 per cent, GDP per capita average annual growth rate was 4.2 per cent, the average annual rate of inflation was 6 per cent, and the percentage of central government expenditure allocated to health was 2 per cent. Most patients do not have health insurance, and have to pay for the tests out of their own pocket. Several hospitals in the government sector in India provide free healthcare service to patients. However, most of these institutions do not have genetic testing services. Hence, at times, the counselee may wish to be tested, but cannot do so because of insufficient funds. A study by Ragothaman et al (2006) on the economic burden of managing Parkinson's disease in India showed that the annual income of nearly half the patients was less than 50,000 rupees (US $ 1,150). Their patients spent nearly one-sixth to more than one-third of their income to buy medicines.

In the West, the guidelines state that for predictive testing, the patient should be counselled, and then given time to digest the information, and the test should be done later. In India, patients come for testing from long distances; therefore, there are difficulties in adhering to pre-test and post-test protocols. It is, therefore, highly impractical to wait after counselling to conduct tests, and genetic testing is usually done on the same day or one to two days after the counselling.

There are no defined community/society forums for adult-onset disorders in India. There is a society for Huntington's disease, and one for spinocerebellar ataxias formed by a patient, but these societies are relatively unknown, and are not accessible to most patients. The decision to test is rarely taken 'voluntarily', but is done under pressure from partners, family and physicians. Due to the joint family system, the individual usually is unable to freely decide whether to be tested or not, and is driven by family and social pressures.

The counsellor

Although the population of India is large, the number of clinical geneticists and genetic counsellors in India is very small, as compared with the volume of patients suffering from common genetic disorders such as Down's syndrome, Duchenne muscular dystrophy (DMD), spinal muscular atrophy (SMA), etc. Therefore, the counselee may not have access to a trained counsellor, and would end up being counselled by a general physician or neurologist without any special training in genetic counselling. Therefore, the counselling may not be appropriate with reference to predictive testing.

In the West, it is standard practice to obtain informed consent prior to obtaining blood samples for any genetic test, but this is not universal practice in India. In our department, we obtain informed consent for predictive testing, but not always for genetic testing in a symptomatic patient. This is because the patient is already symptomatic and has been referred to our lab for a diagnostic test for confirmation.

According to the guidelines established by the International Huntington Association (IHA) and the World Federation of Neurology Research
Group on Huntington's disease (1994), no discrimination of any kind
must result against positively tested individuals. However, in India,
there is stigma attached to any form of illness, handicap or neurological
condition. Indians are very conscious of their status, both social and
economic. This stigmatisation makes it difficult to provide long-term
care for disorders such as Huntington's disease, Parkinson's disease
and spinocerebellar ataxias. Due to the joint family system, the spouse
and the parents, rather than the friends, colleagues and employers, provide psychological and social support.

It happens often that a medical specialist such as a neurologist refers
a patient for predictive testing for HD, without taking a comprehensive
family history or without providing appropriate counselling. In such
cases, the patient and family miss out on a discussion of the pros and
cons of predictive testing, and do not understand the full implications
of the test result. Moreover, psychiatric counselling and referral is not a
routine practice in identifying patients who may be emotionally fragile,
or harbour a psychiatric condition that could be further worsened by
the stress caused by predictive testing. The joint family system does
help them to cope with the result of the genetic test. However, India is
changing rapidly and there is an increasing trend towards nuclear families in cities. Support services for at-risk individuals would be useful,
but these services are lacking in India.

Counselling and genetic testing services in India do not have a follow-up protocol in place to provide support during the post-test stage.
Patients with negative test results are not given due importance during
follow-up, and thus may suffer from untoward post-test reactions.

The international guidelines insist that patient privacy must be
guarded at all times. Clinicians, counsellors or technical staff should
not communicate information concerning the test results to third parties without the permission of the patient/applicant. We do follow this
principle in our centre, and give the test result either to the doctor, or
the patient or someone nominated by the patient. At times, the patient
asks the parents, siblings or other relatives to collect the report.

The genetic laboratory

There are only two or three laboratories in India offering molecular testing for Huntington's disease. Our laboratory carries out the maximum
molecular tests for adult-onset disorders such as Huntington's disease,
spinocerebellar ataxias and familial cancer. Samples therefore are often
sent to these laboratories from places at some distance away. Our laboratory has three trained genetic counsellors attached to it, while the

other two have one each. Since counsellors are not available in remote places, the genetic tests are often performed without the patient having been counselled. However, with most of these patients, the tests are carried out in the presence of some symptoms. The neurologists or the physicians who see these patients often do not advise about testing of other family members. In the event that a patient tests positive for one of these disorders, we do state in our report that 'this result has important implications for the family members', but leave it to the patient or the doctor to inform the other relatives.

At times, the doctor ordering the test is in a different place than the residence of the patient, so that the laboratory is requested to send the report not only to the physician but also to the patient. In such cases, we do advise the patient who tests positive to contact the referring doctor. We have not studied the implications of such a policy, and perhaps it may be better to send the report to the doctor only, and ask the patient to collect the results from the doctor. This would ensure that the patient with a positive test result is given proper counselling by the referring physician.

There is no quality assurance program for molecular genetic testing in India as yet. It is necessary that the professional associations in India constitute an External Quality Assurance Scheme (EQAS) program to ensure the accuracy of the results in the laboratories in India. Efforts are underway to set up EQAS programme in India.

It is our practice to store the DNA sample of the patient, for use in testing the family or for prenatal diagnosis in the future, if requested by the patient. We also store it for research, since we have a clause in the consent form that the sample may be stored for use for research in an anonymous way.

Survey to evaluate the attitude of patients and their families towards the genetic testing

Counsellors and physicians need to be extremely careful when offering predictive genetic tests in India, due to widely differing educational levels, cultural and social beliefs. We faced many such issues when we undertook predictive testing for HD in India. As there are no formal guidelines for predictive testing in India, we decided to evaluate attitudes towards the testing and analyse its implications with respect to the existing social and religious values.

The study was carried out at the Department of Genetic Medicine, Sir Ganga Ram Hospital, New Delhi, India. This is a super-speciality healthcare and research centre. A questionnaire eliciting opinions and attitudes on various personal, social, and present health status, and future healthcare with regard to presymptomatic and prenatal testing for HD, was designed. This questionnaire was then sent out to 35 patients and/or their family members who had tested positive for HD. Thirteen people responded to the questionnaire and participated in the study.

Profile of surveyed subjects

The participants were from different parts of India, with varying religious, social and cultural backgrounds. These participants ranged in age from 26 to 63 years. About 38 per cent were educated to secondary school level; approximately 47 per cent were graduates while 15 per cent had gained professional degrees. A majority of participants (92 per cent) were married. Sixty-seven per cent of married subjects had two children, while 25 per cent had three to four children. None of the children were diagnosed with HD; however, in two cases, the oldest children (aged 5 and 8 years) were presenting symptoms similar to HD as reported by the parents. All the participants were symptomatic when they were tested, and all of them tested positive for the expanded Huntington allele. Three participants (23 per cent) consumed alcohol, and two of these three (67 per cent) reduced their alcohol intake after learning their test results.

The decision to get tested

When asked about the reasons for opting for the genetic test, 85 per cent of the patients said they decided for the test in order to confirm the diagnosis, while 10 per cent were tested as they were interested in prenatal diagnosis in future pregnancies. Another 5 per cent took the test because of anxiety due to a positive family history.

Awareness about the genetic aspects of HD

In 23 per cent of the cases, the positively tested patients were not aware of the risk of HD in their children and siblings, while 8 per cent of the subjects were partially informed and knew about the risk to their children but did not know about the risk to their siblings. This reflects poor counselling and pre-test and post-test guidance about inheritance of the disease. The majority (70 per cent) of the patients, however, were aware of the risk to family members.

The consequences of testing

Testing positive has obvious consequences. Anger, anxiety and depression are all commonly encountered emotions. There is likely to be a period of mourning for the carefree future the person had hoped to enjoy. However, people have different strategies to cope with positive test results. On enquiring about their reaction to the positive genetic test results for HD, 42% of the patients felt relief after knowing the cause of their illness and were glad to be given a chance to plan their future life accordingly. Two of the five patients expressed mixed feelings of relief, grief and isolation from others. However, 38% patients expressed negative emotions such as sadness, grief, shock and depression. Two individuals with positive family history of HD also felt anger at parents and a sense of loss of control.

Sharing test results

About 23% of the individuals had not shared the test result with anyone. About 20% of individuals did not want to communicate test results to their family members and friends, because the children were too young (33%), or they did not want to upset / shock the family (22%). Some (33%) felt that their test result did not concern family members and friends and felt no benefit in communicating results to them. One individual stated that he was not ready to communicate the positive test result to anyone due to the fear of being treated differently. Some of those individuals who tested positive were unaware of any family history of HD. This may be due to secrecy being maintained in the family.

Quality of support from family

On enquiring about the quality of support they received from close friends and family, 33 per cent of individuals rated 'very supportive', 42 per cent marked 'supportive', while 25 per cent marked 'somewhat supportive'. This reflects the need for external support systems and social help for patients and families undergoing predictive testing. There is a dearth of such services in India. However, India's closely-knit family structure has many advantages. The strong bond between the families and the joint family structure help in sharing and providing emotional support for the patients.

Recommending testing to others

Most of the patients (80 per cent) believed in predictive testing and felt that knowing their status was so much better than not knowing at all. A few patients (20 per cent) and their immediate family members decided not to suggest to others in the family to go for predictive HD testing as they felt it would not do them any good, since there is no cure available. About 80 per cent of the participants would recommend testing to other people in the same situation. About 46 per cent of the patients expressed interest in testing their children once they reach an adult age, while 31 per cent would let the children make the decision themselves once they reach adult age. Approximately 15 per cent were against testing their children. One couple, although interested in testing their children aged 3 and 5 years, decided against it after receiving post-test counselling at our centre. One participant was keen to have his two children, both younger than 10 years, tested.

Most individuals (92 per cent) were married, of whom a majority (90 per cent) did not plan to have more children. Most of the subjects (75 per cent) were well past their reproductive age to have more children. Almost one-fourth of subjects did not want to have any more children because of their positive test result.

Effect of positive test result on daily living

A positive test result can affect everyday life in numerous ways. All the participants in the survey were symptomatic for HD (see Table 5.1). In our survey, 15 per cent of the participants who were diagnosed with HD had problems at work once they started showing symptoms of HD. One of the subjects used to be a tailor by profession, and had to discontinue work because of onset of the disease. Another subject who was a teacher stated that she was having trouble socialising, and this also affected her job. One stated that he has to ask for support/help for all daily activities. This has made him dependent on the family for his daily personal needs as well. Most also felt that the positive test had altered their reproductive choices.

Table 5.1   *Clinical manifestations of HD in the 13 individuals participating in the Survey*

Clinical symptoms	No.	% (approx.)
Involuntary movements	11	85
Memory affected	10	77
Impaired concentration	11	85
Speech affected	9	69
Sleep affected	7	54
Significant weight loss	5	39
Mild to moderate depression	4	31
Difficulty in writing	11	85
Difficulty in holding objects	8	62
Difficulty in walking straight	6	46
Difficulty in eating/swallowing	7	54

Family history

All of the subjects had at least one affected family member and seven subjects had two or more affected family members. In spite of having a prominent positive family history of HD, only three out of thirteen of these people had relatives who got tested. In 46 per cent, the disease was inherited maternally, and in 54 per cent of cases inherited from the paternal side. None of them was a de novo case arising from new mutations.

Attitude towards prenatal testing

When we enquired about their interest in prenatal testing, almost half of the subjects answered affirmatively, while a quarter decided against prenatal testing in future pregnancies. One subject was undecided on the topic. If, hypothetically speaking, the foetus is found to have the defective HD gene during prenatal diagnosis, 86 per cent of the subjects said they would opt for abortion, and, surprisingly, one of them said that he would want the pregnancy to continue, despite having an affected parent and two affected maternal uncles. This could be because of personal choice, or because it was a hypothetical situation and he would probably decide otherwise if he faced the situation in reality. It could also be because of religious beliefs, though we do have couples opting for prenatal diagnosis of other genetic disorders even though their religion does not permit abortions.

Effect of positive result on future plans

In the present survey, all but one of the subjects stated that positive results would impact their life decisions. One woman, with an affected parent, was very relieved and felt solace in knowing the 'cause' of her symptoms. According to her, this was 'one step to improving her quality of life, if not more.' One subject also expressed that he was glad to receive his results, as living in uncertainty was very difficult. He felt stronger and bolder to face the consequences of HD now. For some, ambiguity about their genetic disease status constituted an obstacle in their lives and prevented them from living happily. Testing eliminated these hindrances and helped them to live proactively and make significant changes in their daily outlook toward life. None of the participants regretted undergoing testing.

Discussion: predictive genetic testing in India

The survey has highlighted some issues with regard to the way counselling is provided to individuals undergoing genetic testing for Huntington's disease or other adult-onset diseases in India. The study subjects
had many questions and fears about their illness, interpretation of test
results and its impact on family members, and psychological and social
support. Some subjects requested more information about the disease
and about the risk to their children. Others enquired about the availability of a cure or treatment. Nagaraja, Jain and Muthane (2006), who studied the attitudes of different groups of Indian people towards presymptomatic testing for HD, also made similar observations. It is thus
essential to understand the concerns of family members at risk for HD
and to ensure that genetic counsellors, physicians and family address
them adequately.

No matter how much an individual prepares for a positive result, he
or she is never prepared enough. There is an immediate feeling of
shock, a moment of crying, followed by a sense of relief to finally know
the results, and not having to question oneself any longer, relief that
now they can focus on what needs to be done, even with a positive result. As long as they know what they are facing, they can fight it. These
individuals learn to appreciate their time and ability to do things. They
learn that staying healthy and as stress-free as possible is the best way
to deal with the disorder or disease they will suffer from in the future.
They find happiness in family and friends. Quoting one such proactive
patient, 'When life gives you lemons, you don't just make lemonade;
you plant the seeds and make trees grow.' Similar reactions were observed in our study, as 42 per cent of the subjects felt relief, although
38 per cent had negative emotions after the test.

Individuals who test positive may avoid visiting their family members
who are dealing with the disease themselves, mainly because it is difficult to be seeing into your own future from up close. HD becomes
more real then. Sometimes, though, the family members can help an
individual to cope with the results, and motivate them to face the disease proactively. One important observation in our survey was that most
patients obtained good family support after a positive test result. Some
individuals often enter the 'fundraising phase', mostly consisting of voluntary service to people affected with the dreaded disease, and getting
involved in raising money for a cure for HD. In one family, the husband built a special home and dedicated it to people with Huntington's
disease. This is, of course, a very healthy way of dealing with a positive
result.

All thirteen of our participants in the study had tested positive;
hence, we were not able to record the reactions after a negative test re-

sult on the subjects in the survey. However, based on our experience with families with Huntington's disease, we noted that many feel hesitant about celebrating their negative test results, when other family members have not been equally fortunate. Psychiatric counselling should be a routine practice in patients who are emotionally fragile or have psychiatric symptoms because their condition could be further worsened by the stress caused by predictive testing.

Some individuals start exploring and learning about the disease to prepare themselves for a positive result, because all their life they think that they will develop HD. The reactions of these individuals can be very unpredictable if they test negative, especially when they have affected family members. After experiencing an immediate relief from the knowledge that they are now not at risk of the disease, they feel complex emotions, partly because they feel guilty that they escaped the disease while other family members suffer from it. Even though friends and family may want to celebrate the news, the individual in question may go into withdrawal and feel grief. To put it in other words, one individual described this feeling like a car crash in which her mother and brothers were severely injured and now have a very short life, but she herself was unhurt and got to live.

Sometimes survivor's guilt causes people to contribute to providing support and care for others affected with the disease. They need time to assimilate the results; it takes a while to stop watching for symptoms and it is common for those who test negative to wonder if a mistake was made with the test. They are offered a repeat sampling and re-testing for reassurance. Such individuals will need psychiatric counselling to come to terms with a lot of issues, because till now they were assuming HD to be the cause of all their problems, and suddenly find that they were not actually due to HD as they tested negative. They will now have to learn to deal with themselves without having HD to blame. Thus, in spite of a negative test result, such individuals go through difficult times and often require psychiatric counselling.

In India, the decision to test is rarely taken 'voluntarily', and under pressure from partners, family and physicians. There is an unquestionable faith in Indian families that the decision taken by the parents for their children is for their best benefit. Often, partners or spouses may want someone to be tested, because of joint decisions that will be made about marriage, having children, taking financial risks, etc. (Nagaraja et al 2006). The individual usually is unable to decide freely whether to be tested or not and is driven by family and social pressure. People unfamiliar with HD, such as friends and colleagues, may be surprised if an at-risk individual does not want to get tested. This is because they have not thought through the implications of learning that one might develop a disease for which there is no cure as yet. Individuals who opt against predictive testing usually do not want to give up hope that they do not carry the defective HD gene. Some individuals, who are planning a family, opt for predictive testing so that they can avoid passing on the disease to their children through prenatal diagnosis or preimplantation genetic diagnosis.

Indian families are usually close-knit and interdependent for their needs. In such a scenario, when one family member wants to get tested, the other members may feel strongly against it, as according to them, his or her status will reflect on their own status, which they are not ready to cope with. A positive test result can bring about panic and restlessness in one's family members concerning the risk to themselves and their children.

Although the joint family system in India has the disadvantage of restricting personal freedom of action, it has the major advantage of providing genuine support to the individual to cope with the adverse effects of a positive result in those opting for predictive genetic testing. It is thus apparent that the regulations and practices that should govern and guide predictive testing differ among different cultures. However, India is changing rapidly and there is now an increasing trend towards nuclear families, associated with modernity. Support services, either hospital-based or through patient's societies, can offer tremendous help to affected families and information for at-risk family members. There are very few societies for adult-onset disorders in India. Many more such societies are required to furnish support to patients and for those undergoing predictive testing.

The present survey revealed that performing the test provided relief from uncertainty in 42 per cent of the subjects. However, the awareness about the disease was very poor, highlighting the need to provide more information to patients with the disease. A significant number did not share the information about the positive test with other family members partly because they did not want to upset them. The majority of subjects would recommend testing to other relatives. Another significant finding was that almost half would favour prenatal diagnosis of the disease to avoid inflicting the disease on the children, while the others were indifferent to the issue as they were beyond the reproductive stage.

The survey established the fact that individual autonomy was less important than the family decision. Arrangements for pre- and post-test counselling need to be addressed in India. Equal availability of services for molecular testing assumes great importance in all developing countries, so that the poor may also access these facilities. Overall, the survey revealed that predictive testing for HD improved the psychological well-being of at-risk individuals; however, proper counselling protocols need to be in place. Most individuals who receive a 'normal' result improved psychological health, while the individuals who knew they were at increased risk after the result did not respond in the catastrophic manner that one might expect.

In India, most people at risk do not go for predictive testing because of lack of knowledge about the disease and its transmission. Although there is shortage of genetic counsellors, nevertheless genetic counselling is important before as well as after testing, to help the people to cope with the situation arising from the results. Genetic counselling is also important to parents whose children are under eighteen, as it would be advisable to postpone genetic testing until the children grow up and can take independent decisions. This should continue until a therapy is developed to halt or alter the course of the disease in those carrying the mutant gene. The joint family system is a positive feature in Indian society, as it provides psychological support to those found to have a positive result. Hopefully, as the awareness about the disease spreads, strong support organisations would be developed to provide information, and help to those who have the disease and those who are at risk of inheriting the disease.

6 How Japanese Women Describe Their Experiences of Prenatal Testing

Azumi Tsuge

Introduction

Japan is one of the countries where ultrasound examination during pregnancy is conducted very frequently. Yet the frequency of maternal serum screening tests and/or amniocentesis in Japan is relatively low (Sagou, Okuyama & Kawane 2002). These phenomena result from historical and current socio-cultural influences, which are the subject of exploration in this chapter.

In this chapter, I describe the reasons why pregnant women do or do not undergo prenatal testing in Japan by presenting the results of our research project on 'Women's Experiences of Pregnancies and Prenatal Tests' (Tsuge, Ishiguro & Sugano 2005). In a period covering most of the last half of the twentieth century, Japan, under the Eugenic Protection Law, limited the right of disabled people to have children (Ichinokawa, Kato & Tsuge 1996; Saito 2002). Partly as a response to this, Japan also has an ongoing history of the disabled rights movement severely criticising prenatal testing, such as amniocentesis, as a form of eugenics, for having the test is perceived as a eugenic practice, encouraging selective abortion when the test result is undesirable.

As medical technologies have developed in the last three decades, the number of women who undergo prenatal tests has increased greatly. However, both women and gynaecologists tend to avoid disclosure of the procedures, to avoid criticism for discrimination against disabled people. The situation is different from what some American scholars show about prenatal testing in the US (Rothman 1993; Rothenberg & Thomson 1994; Rapp 1999). As very few social research studies about women's views on prenatal tests have been conducted in Japan, we decided to undertake research to clarify the situation of prenatal testing. In 2003, we conducted questionnaire-based research regarding women's experiences with their pregnancies and prenatal testing in Tokyo. Of the nine hundred copies of the questionnaire distributed to women with at least one child aged five or under, 382 completed sheets were re-

turned anonymously by mail, giving us a response rate of 42.4 per cent.
Three hundred and seventy-five valid responses were used in our analysis. The 375 women reported that they experienced 714 pregnancies in
total over the last ten years, which resulted in the birth of 550 children
(Tsuge, Ishiguro & Sugano 2005).

Why women undergo ultrasound examinations

In Japan, ultrasound examination during maternity care is very common.
In the US, according to the Centers for Disease Control and Prevention
(CDC) (2005: 2), 67 per cent of women who had live births received ul-
trasound tests in 2003 (cf. 47.6 per cent in 1989, 60 per cent in 1993).

In our results, ninety-nine per cent of the women underwent ultrasound exams during the prenatal period. Many of them had exams
every time they went to see their obstetrician or gynaecologist ('obstetrician' from here onwards), while some had only a few or several ultra-
sounds during the period. It is difficult to say exactly how many times
women have the tests during a pregnancy because each obstetrician has
a different policy about the advisable frequency of ultrasound that pregnant women should undergo. In fact, there are no guidelines about the
frequency of the use of the test in Japan. All obstetrician clinics have ultrasound scanners, which the doctors routinely use. Many doctors are
not even concerned about the risks of ultrasound exams or the cost, but
some doctors are concerned about its risks to pregnant women and
their foetuses.

Many women obtained information about ultrasound exams not from
medical doctors, but from magazines. Only 24 per cent of the women
surveyed responded that they are informed about the purpose, methods
and/or risks of ultrasound exams. Furthermore, only 8 per cent of them
were asked by their physician if they wanted a scan.

In the following, I present the narratives of these women in order to
arrive at a better understanding of factors that have strongly affected
these women in their decision-making. They described why they
decided to undergo the exams as follows:
– It was routine to have the test.
– I just followed the doctor's orders.
– I didn't know if I could decline the test.

Otherwise, they emphasised the benefits to them of undergoing the ultrasound test.
– I enjoyed seeing my baby every time I went to the doctor. I was able
  to show the pictures to my parents and mother-in-law. Then they
  enjoyed them too.

- Even though I had felt uncomfortable during the transvaginal ultrasound test, it made me more aware of the mother's role when I was in danger of miscarrying. I welcomed the chance to have the test as the only way to know my child's condition in the early stage of pregnancy.
- I suppose it also made my husband more aware of his new family role.

Many of the women who enjoyed 'seeing their babies' do not recognise that ultrasound testing is also used to confirm if their foetus has a problem and, if it does, to choose whether to keep their pregnancy or not. Not only women, but also some medical doctors, seem to be unaware of what they can find out by the use of ultrasound testing and how they should deal with unexpected and unwelcome information about the foetus. As a result of ultrasound exams, some women reported that unexpected information about their foetus, such as anencephaly, which shows the probability of Down's syndrome, caused them severe shock.

- In the sixth month of my second pregnancy, my baby was diagnosed as a deformed (anencephalic) baby. Therefore, I had to make the very tough decision of having induced abortion. To be honest, ultrasound testing may not work as a complete safeguard to support pregnant women until their delivery; however, if you decided to undergo a test, you would still feel the sense of relief. Also, medical specialists could discover serious problems and detect, to some degree, the baby's condition, and they should be able to provide appropriate advice.
- My doctor noticed that the foetus had tumidity [nuchal translucency], due to a chromosomal aberration. I was very shocked to hear that and I was depressed and cried during the last part of the pregnancy. But, in fact, the baby was perfectly healthy after having an operation for tumidity. I don't think the doctor's information was appropriate. I fear that medical technology used unthinkingly gives us more information than we can use.

However, it does not provide a simple resolution just to inform women of the possibility that they could find an undesirable condition in their foetus. For instance, a few women describe their dilemma regarding possible ultrasound tests because they were deeply aware that the ultrasound test could present them with some very serious problems.

- I thought that ultrasound testing was supposed to 'discriminate' the healthy foetus from defect ones, but I could not resist looking at the picture. I had to try not to think about the possibility of fetal abnormalities. I don't know what 'discriminate' means here.

– I felt a dilemma between suffering through the pregnancy with an abnormal foetus and terminating the pregnancy. At the same time I did not know if any of the abnormalities would be treatable. At last I decided to have the test. The ultrasound found nothing abnormal. But, in fact, the baby was malformed.

We asked the women who had decided to perform their ultrasound examination. Forty percent (151 cases) replied that the doctor had, but 26 per cent (96 cases) chose 'I did', and 25 per cent (94 cases) chose 'the doctor and I did'. Interestingly, only 34 out of 96 women who chose 'I did' were informed about the exams. It means that a considerable number of them think that they participated in the decision-making without actually having accurate information on it.

On the basis of the response for the open-ended question, we understand the factors of influence on this phenomenon as follows:

– The women assume they have enough information about the ultrasound exam from magazines, their friends or sisters who have had babies, or their own experiences, even though the information is skewed or inaccurate.
– They aspire to 'see their babies' through the ultrasound device not only for their peace of mind but also for fun. The picture of the foetus is probably a tool for inspiring paternal love and for establishing good relationships between couples and their parents.
– They suppose that the exam is routine because doctors do not give them information and do not ask their consent to do it, and thus they suppose it must be safe and useful.

When women make the decision of undergoing maternal serum screening or amniocentesis, women prepare themselves in case any fetal abnormalities are detected. In contrast, an ultrasound exam is frequently conducted without being recognised as a prenatal examination. As a result, an enjoyable occasion to see the foetus could suddenly turn out to be a test that informs the parents of some abnormality, raising the question of whether the pregnancy should be continued or not.

Historical background of prenatal testing

Here, I will present the historical background to prenatal testing and attitudes to induced abortion in Japan, because I believe that this is critical for accurately interpreting and understanding the experience and opinions of many women who participated in our survey and interviews regarding prenatal testing.

In Japan, maternal serum screening and amniocentesis are not prevalent, even though these prenatal tests were introduced into Japan as early as the 1950s and 1960s, while ultrasound screening is widely used. Some factors behind this trend include discussions held since the 1970s regarding the violated rights of disabled people to live and to be born, accompanying the increase of prenatal testing and the resulting selective abortion. This trend was ideologically supported by the movement of disabled people and feminists against the Eugenic Protection Law, in effect until 1996 (e.g. Ogino 2004; Kato 2005).

Japan explicitly had eugenics policies during the Pacific War. It coerced disabled people into not having children by employing various eugenic means. This law was enforced in 1948 when Japan was recovering from the defeat of World War II, following the lines of the National Eugenic Law promulgated in 1941. In this period, eugenic policies were applied even to family planning in many countries. It is not surprising then that the Japanese new 'liberal and left-wing' government, and not a government associated with imperialism and militarism, applied a eugenic policy in the late 1940s and 1950s. Although the law was known as a way to legalise induced abortion and sterilisation, the reality was that it was enacted for the purpose of controlling the 'quantity and the quality of the population'. At the same time, the illegality of abortion was retained as stipulated in the Penal Code, which was enacted in 1880 and revised in 1907. It implied that induced abortion was not permitted as a right of women to make a choice, but as a means of population control (Matsubara 2002).

In 1950, economic conditions were identified as a valid prerequisite for administering the law, with the result that induced abortion became the most common method for promoting family planning. As a result, over one million induced abortions were conducted and officially reported for the year 1950, giving rise to the view that the method of induced abortion could increase the effect of the population control policy. As induced abortion was not then legal in the US and many European countries, Japan was ridiculed as 'abortion heaven'. Since then, different types of contraception have been used, and the number of abortions has declined. At the same time, the total fertility rate also began to decline.

In 1972, the anti-abortion lobby submitted a revised bill to the Diet. In addition to the removal of the economic reasons clause, it proposed to allow abortion if the foetus was suspected of having a serious mental or physical defect, and also to advise Japanese women to give birth to their first child at a 'suitable age'. While aimed at increasing fertility rates, the bill simultaneously advocated that eugenically 'undesirable' children should not be born.

Ogino (2004), a specialist on the history of Japanese population policy and women's reproductive rights, summarised the contention of the people-with-disability movement as follows:

> They argued that social tolerance for killing a disabled foetus is synonymous with saying to those living with disability, 'You are not supposed to exist in this world. You'd better die.' At the same time, they questioned the fundamental validity of abortion sanctioned by the Eugenic Protection Law and criticised the claim that abortion was a woman's right to choose, saying that this was nothing but a 'healthy person's egoism' and that women were taking part in sustaining discrimination against the disabled. Thus, two socially marginalised groups, women and people with disabilities, were placed in awkward confrontation in connection with the Eugenic Protection Law.

Introducing the bill also caused constant conflict between the women's movement and groups of disabled people, both of which are marginalised groups in Japan. The issue at stake focused especially on the right of women to choose induced abortion.

Attitudes to 'selective abortion'

According to official statistics in Japan, the number of induced abortions in 2005 exceeded 289,000 cases. This is a significant number, considering the fact that the number of live births each year is approximately 1.1 million, and that probably not all induced abortions are reported. However, for over a century, criminal law has contained a provision for prohibiting abortion under pronatalism. In 1948, induced abortion was enforced only under narrow conditions, such as the health concerns for the pregnant woman, eugenic reasons including genetic diseases of the pregnant woman and/or her spouse, and pregnancy due to sexual assault (e.g. Norgren 2001).

Currently, induced abortion is allowed with approval from the spouse only if the pregnancy period is less than 22 weeks. However, because at the time the use of prenatal testing could not be foreseen, the induced abortion of a severely impaired foetus was not included. Such a condition is now categorised as leading to health or financial conditions so as to legally allow its abortion. In fact, over 90 per cent of induced abortions are reported as conducted due to 'financial conditions', which indicates that women are in a situation where they could virtually obtain abortion on demand.

At the same time, many women advocating reproductive freedom were both disturbed and moved by the criticism of disabled people. While they fully recognised the vital importance and necessity of legal abortion for women's lives, they realised at the same time that their claim to have a right to abortion under the present state of the law could be easily exploited and used in such a way as to eliminate the right of the disabled.

Ogino (2004) cites the following words of Tanaka, one of the most well-known figures of the Japanese women's liberation movement in the 1970s, which reflect the peculiar dilemma with which Japanese feminists were confronted:

> Women's liberationists in Europe and America claim for the freedom of and right to abortion, because they primarily seek liberation from the religious morals such as Catholicism. In Japan, however, induced abortion has been legalised since 1948, though not in a quite satisfactory manner. We Japanese women have not been denied abortion by religious morals, but have resorted to abortion because we think that we should not give birth under inauspicious circumstances we live in, and in doing so have contributed to increasing corporate benefits. We cannot and dare not say so readily that abortion is our right. ... If we do not perceive our pain in conducting forced infanticide and keep resorting to abortion for the reason that there is no way to escape from society, we will inevitably be caught up in the stink of this efficiency-oriented, dog-eat-dog world that attaches higher value to the production of automobiles than to children's lives. (Tanaka 1973: 4)

I would like to introduce comments by Yonezu, a feminist activist with a disability who fought against the revision of the Eugenic Protection Law in the 1970s and 1980s, and who asserts that selective abortion after prenatal screening should not be considered a 'woman's reproductive right':

> Abortion after prenatal screening is conducted not because the pregnancy itself is unwanted but in the expectation of having a baby. It is a challenge to decide whether to welcome that child or not, depending on the existence or non-existence of defects. I think that a foetus is neither an independent life nor a part of the woman's body. It is not the same as a person after birth, but it has a potentially to become one. Just as discrimination against a living human being for her or his attributes is wrong, so is discrimination against a foetus. (...) Notwithstanding the fact that it

is society's unkindness to people with disabilities that makes the lives of disabled persons difficult, proponents of prenatal diagnosis pretend that there is no such liability and try to induce women to select their children. The designation of such selection as a woman's 'right' to be practised at her own responsibility actually is a new trend of eugenics, and is nothing but an infringement of women's reproductive rights. (Yonezu 2002: 17-18)

Social scientist Masae Kato conducted research regarding 'rights' in the Japanese women's movement and pointed out the issue of 'right' in local context. She states that the meaning of 'right' in a women's movement in one geographical area might differ from the meaning in other areas. This should not be a problem, because 'right' needs to be localised anyway, and for women in the world to unite together it is important to share experiences about the practice of rights in their activities (Kato 2005: 8).

In 1996, the law was revised as the Maternal Protection Law, which deals with induced abortion and sterilisation, deleting all clauses that could be interpreted as ideologically eugenic. This can be attributed to the disabled people and feminist movement, and the change of citizens' views toward the rights of disabled people.

The current situation on maternal serum screening and amniocentesis

There are no official statistics about the maternal serum screening test and amniocentesis in Japan, but there are a few reliable nationwide survey reports about them (Sagou et al 2002). As shown in Table 6.1, the number of maternal serum screening tests was 21,000 cases in 1998, but 15,900 in 2000. According to Sato, who is a leading specialist on prenatal testing in Japan, the number of triple marker tests conducted in the United States is about 167 times that of Japan, and the frequency of amniocentesis in Germany is more than ten times that of Japan (Sato 1999). As for the number of amniocentesis tests, the annual total is ap-

Table 6.1 *The annual number of maternal serum marker screening tests and amniocentesis in Japan, 1998-2000*

Year	1998	1999	2000
Maternal serum marker screening	21,708	18,312	15,927
Amniocentesis	10,419	10,516	10,627

Source: Sagou, H. et al 2002

proximately 10,000 cases. This number is equivalent to less than 1 per cent of all pregnancy cases per year from 1998 to 2000. The US National Vital Statistics Reports, compiled by the CDC, reported 'the overall rate for amniocentesis continued to decrease. The amniocentesis rate was 1.7 per cent of all live births in 2003, down from 1.9 per cent in 2002 and 3.2 per cent in 1989. This continuing downturn may reflect increased use of non-invasive screening tests in place of amniocentesis (e.g. ultrasound and measurement of serum markers)' (Centers for Disease Control and Prevention 2005: 2).

In 1999, a working committee on the maternal serum screening test, the Japanese Ministry of Health and Welfare, published its views on the maternal serum screening test for the purpose of regulating and countering the increasing popularity of the screening. The test is reported to have the following distinctions and problems:
- There is a tendency for pregnant women to have this test without enough knowledge of what is involved and its consequences.
- Pregnant women misunderstand or become anxious about the result, which shows only probability, not certainty.
- There is concern about this test being used for the mass screening of fetal diseases because it is easy to use.

Therefore, it continues to be the policy that medical doctors are not required to actively inform pregnant women of the existence of this test. In addition, medical doctors should not recommend having the test, and companies should not make and distribute documents to canvass clients for this test. However, when a pregnant woman asks either a medical doctor or a company to explain about the test, they are obliged to inform her about it. The effect of these guidelines was a rapid decline in the number of tests, as Table 6.1 shows.

Why did the working committee conclude that 'medical doctors do not need to inform pregnant women about the maternal serum marker screening test'? First, it became clear that there were some cases in which women misunderstood the test results, which led to unnecessarily induced abortion without having prior amniocentesis. Secondly, a news documentary reported about a company that intended to recommend this test strongly in its advertisement campaign for commercial gain. Distinctly, even though it does not spell it out explicitly, the guideline clearly aims for medical doctors to avoid being sued for 'wrongful birth'.

In such circumstances, there seems to be no uniformity of information available to pregnant women. While some of them do not know anything about the prenatal tests, others receive information from their friends or family, although it is not always accurate. The mass media are also a source of information for pregnant women, although it is not as thorough as it could be.

Attitudes toward the maternal serum screening test and amniocentesis

Going back to the results of the project, a discussion follows on some of the responses to our questionnaire regarding the maternal serum screening test and amniocentesis. In response to our questionnaire, 237 women out of 375 answered that they knew only 'a little' about maternal serum screening during their pregnancy, but 138 women answered that they did not know about it at all. Only 43 women out of 237 answered that they had undergone the test.

Most of these women who took the maternal serum screening test clearly understood the nature of this test because of valuable information supplied by doctors as well as by friends who had already taken these tests. However, a few women who underwent maternal serum screening did not understand its purpose, its methods and the correct interpretation of the results. Furthermore, many of the women who did not take this test made their decision while depending on ambiguous and/or incorrect information.

Concerning amniocentesis, 335 women (89 per cent) answered that they knew about the test and 40 (11 per cent) answered they didn't know about it at all. The following analysis was carried out for the 335 cases.

We asked whether doctors or other medical staff had explained amniocentesis testing. Only 94 women (28 per cent) could confirm that the doctor had followed informed consent procedures, but 66 per cent of the women could not. The mean age of the informed group is about 34 years old; for the uninformed group it is 31 years old. Thus, it can be said that doctors choose who they inform about the test based on the pregnant woman's age. When asked, 'Did your doctor ask whether you wanted to undergo an amniocentesis test?", 23 per cent reported 'Yes' and 72 per cent reported 'No'.

Bearing in mind that the ratio of the women undergoing informed consent procedures for ultrasound examination was 24 per cent, the difference in the ratio of those who were fully aware of the meaning and significance of the ultrasound and amniocentesis was not great. However, there is a big difference in the attitudes of the women toward having the test. Most women had an ultrasound test even if they were not informed about the test, but most women who were uninformed about amniocentesis did not have it. As a result, only 22 underwent amniocentesis.

Reasons for having or not having amniocentesis

Here, I discuss some reasons for having the test, put forward by 18 out of the 22 women who underwent amniocentesis, when responding to an open-ended question about it. Nine out of sixteen said being over 35 years old was the reason for having the test. Four of the women who were under 34 years old responded that they were motivated by the results of the maternal serum screening test, which showed them to be at 'high risk'. Six out of the 22 women reported that they wanted to know the condition of the foetus because they felt anxious about their pregnancies. Two of them stated that they wanted to know the condition in order to prepare for having a child with an abnormality, not for potentially having a abortion. Three out of 22 reported that they thought it natural to have the test or that the doctor had recommended having the test. One of them answered that she had had the test in a foreign country. She stated that many women had the test in the country where she stayed.

– Looking back at the experience, it frightens me. But I felt conflicted about having a disabled child. Although I understand the meaning of 'equality' and 'dignity of life' in my mind, I did not want to bear a child with a disability. I can't tell anyone that I had this test because of feeling guilty even after I gave birth.
– I had a strange feeling, as I realised what was found by the test. I also felt guilty about making the decision about life or death connected with having an abortion because of foetal abnormality.
– I heard about a horrible experience about amniocentesis from my friend. She had a miscarriage right after having amniocentesis, and the foetus did not have Down's syndrome. I have sympathy for those who worry about having children with a disability because of the social discrimination against disabled people.

It is clear that conflicting feelings of guilt and worry play an important role in deciding whether or not to undergo amniocentesis.

Next, I would like to explain the reasons for not having the test by using data from the 147 out of 283 women who responded to the open-ended question on this topic. Sixty-one women pointed out the risks accompanying the test, such as miscarriage, harming the foetus, and injuring the mother. Forty-six women reported that they thought that they did not need to undergo the test because of their age or their health condition.

– I was reluctant to terminate the life that I had started at last, in this pregnancy ... before it came. I wonder, you cannot help it, if there is a physical reason for the foetus being abnormal, but I am very reluctant to have amniocentesis. Because I think it is like denying the whole personality of the child.

Interestingly enough, 38 women reported that the doctor did not provide information about amniocentesis so they believed that they did not need it. In addition, 15 women reported that the doctor had not recommended the test.

- I wondered if I would need to have amniocentesis once. But I didn't do it because my doctor hadn't discussed it with me.
- I worried about the foetus [disability] a lot during my first pregnancy, so I decided to consult friends, my sister, husband, and others. As I asked my doctor about amniocentesis, he said that I may not need to have the test, but ... I did not have it, as I believed my doctor's view. When I got pregnant with my second child, I asked another doctor about the test. He said that there is a test to check the condition of the foetus, but ... I understood the doctor didn't advise me to have it. Both children don't have any problem with their health. I assume I would have had the test if the doctor had recommended having it.

Thirty women reported that they had decided to continue the pregnancy even if the baby had an abnormality, so they thought that they did not need the test. Seventeen women reported that they could not decide what they would do if the test showed any problem.

- I did not waver about not having amniocentesis in the beginning of my pregnancy. I did not have it. I would have had the test if it had been possible to treat any problem detected. I assume that I would have spent the pregnancy period being gloomy if I had known there was something wrong with my child through having amniocentesis, because I had decided not to have an abortion.
- I decided not to have amniocentesis, together with my partner. But it is horrible to imagine how I would have behaved, what conflict I would have experienced, if I had known about an abnormality of the foetus through the test.
- I took the maternal serum screening test, and it showed high risk. I was informed about amniocentesis and I had it. The result showed that my foetus did not have a problem. I was relieved to hear it. Actually, I was left with a bad taste in my mouth because I had not been able to make a decision before I heard the test result. I had considered for a long time seriously what I should do if I got a bad result. During my second pregnancy, I remember that I was really relieved when I received the negative [low risk] result of the maternal serum screening test.

On the basis of the results and views above, below I will summarise the factors that have affected the process of decision-making on prenatal testing, which is distinctive of the attitude and cognition to prenatal testing of women in Japan.

First, many women do not recognise that the ultrasound test is also a part of prenatal tests. They enjoy seeing pictures of their foetus and emphasise the importance of the test. Only a few are aware that an ultrasound test is also a prenatal test, which may force a woman to make a decision whether to give birth or terminate pregnancy. Second, with regard to maternal serum screening and amniocentesis, women clearly demonstrate their conflicting feelings of guilt and worry when making decisions about their pregnancy. Several women described their critique of prenatal tests explicitly, calling it 'discrimination against foetuses with a disability', even though they did not object to other women's choice to have an abortion. Third, many women reported that they did not have maternal serum screening and amniocentesis, because their doctors did not explain it to them. In other words, they believed that they did not need prenatal tests. Although some doctors emphasise that it is the women's choice to have the test or not, many women still appear to expect and rely upon the doctor's paternalistic role. Finally, several women reported that they had already decided to continue the pregnancy even if the baby had an abnormality, so they thought that they did not need the test. Some women reported that they worried about deciding what they would do if the test indicated any problem. These responses showed that women preferred not to know about the condition of the foetus rather than to have a hard time making a decision after undergoing prenatal tests. This attitude seems to strongly influence the choice of women in Japan to refuse a prenatal test.

Discussion

Even though the women enjoyed seeing their 'babies' and they reported that while the image of the foetus had encouraged them to go through ultrasound exams, it might cause problems to them as well. In fact, a few women reported that the unexpected information about their foetus by ultrasound exam, such as anencephaly or a boil, which indicates the probability of Down's syndrome, caused them severe shock. I think that both the doctors and the pregnant women should be aware of the issues involved when undergoing ultrasound examination.

A comparison of the research results between ultrasound testing and amniocentesis shows that women tend to believe that 'they made the decision' to have a test when they were asked for their consent or will by their doctor. However, even when they were not asked for their consent or will and they assumed that it was only a routine test, many of them answered that 'they made the decision' to undergo the test.

I believe that they assumed they had enough information about the ultrasound test to make a decision, not necessarily as a result of the doctor's advice, but because they had read about it in the media. Also, their positive impression of the test affected their awareness of having made the decision. The research results also show, however, that many women also rely on their doctor's information and advice about having tests.

Furthermore, the phenomenon of women saying that they made pre-natal decisions is a new dimension of the issue in Japan. Previously, women were used to referring prenatal medical decisions to their part-ners or parents-in-law for fear that they would be blamed for doing the wrong thing. Recently, however, I find the question of 'who makes the decision' itself is changing. The expression 'self-determination' is be-coming pervasive in many fields in Japan; that is, women are starting to admit to wanting to take responsibility for making their own decisions.

This self-determination also influences the way in which doctors choose to present or not present prenatal testing to their patients. In the case of ultrasound, the traditional 'good' (paternalistic) doctor uses prenatal testing only when 'needed' and without explanation. The 'new-style' doctor, however, sees ultrasound testing as an 'added-value' ser-vice that should be offered to all patients or clients. Especially in the case of amniocentesis, many women reported that the reason for them not to have the test was that the doctor did not discuss it with them, and thus they thought the test was not necessary. This can be explained by residual paternalism. Although some doctors emphasised that it was the patient's choice to have the test or not, many women expect and rely upon the doctor's paternalistic role.

Because of the 1970s disability rights movement in Japan, some wo-men and their partners, as well as some doctors, believe that amnio-centesis somewhat discriminates against disabled people. Thus, many respondents felt that amniocentesis was immoral, and they had diffi-culty making a choice. However, few people are aware that an ultra-sound test is also a prenatal test, sometimes with the same issues.

Table 6.2 shows most women who took the maternal serum screen-ing tests and/or amniocentesis gave informed consent. Their responses to the question also show that they understood the nature of these tests because of valuable information supplied by doctors, as well as by friends who had already taken these tests. However, some women who took the maternal serum screening test did not correctly understand the meaning of the result. Furthermore, many women who did not take these tests made their decisions while depending on ambiguous and/or wrong information.

Table 6.2 *Correlations among those tested, informed consent/no informed consent from doctors, and age (n=305)*

	Tested (22)		Not tested (283)	
	Under 34 years old	Over 35 years old	Under 34 years old	Over 35 years old
Given informed consent	4	16	34	39
No informed consent	2	0	122	88

The 'No Answer' cases are deleted

One typical answer from women who did not undergo the tests and had inadequate information was that they had judged that they did not need the tests simply because their doctors did not provide them with information. The project results show that the main reason for not taking the test was because the mother was young and healthy. This led them to believe that, in turn, their baby would not have any problems.

Some responded that they were prepared to nurture disabled children and/or that they did not consider having an abortion even in case of the unexpected. Overall, the most frequent explanation for not taking the tests was that it was difficult for them to make a decision based on the tests, so they avoided them.

I would like to point out that women's attitudes toward prenatal testing in Japan are different from those in North America, where people attach higher value to 'choice'. In Japan, women tend to say that 'they made a decision' in an easy case. Yet they avoid choosing in cases they perceive as difficult, such as whether or not to have amniocentesis and whether to terminate pregnancy or to give birth. This attitude appears to be an important factor for explaining the current situation concerning prenatal testing in Japan.

Acknowledgement

This project was fully funded by a Japanese Grant-in-Aid for Scientific Research, 2003-2005. I would like to express my sincere thanks to Ms S. Sugano, MA, and Ms M. Ishiguro as collaborators in the research project, 'Women's Experience of Pregnancies and Prenatal Testing in Japan'.

7 Cultural Notions of Disability in Japan: Their Influence on Prenatal Testing

Masae Kato

A number of socio-cultural factors influence individuals' decision-making whether to undertake prenatal testing to check the health of a foetus, such as the price of the test and the healthcare system, as well as advice from medical professionals (Sleeboom-Faulkner 2004b). Among all these factors, this chapter focuses on the cultural concept of disabilities in Japan as an influential factor for deciding whether to undertake prenatal screening.

Not surprisingly, different social groups and individuals have different views on disability. Looking at public debates in Japan about the pros and cons for the practice of prenatal testing, the following groups can be raised as influential in formulating public debates on regulating prenatal testing in Japan: medical associations, the women's reproductive health movement and the disabled people's movement.

The disabled people's movements tend to oppose the practice of prenatal testing. As reproductive genetic technologies seek to find anomalies in foetuses, and as most of positive test results lead to termination of pregnancy,[1] they contend that the technologies aim at eradicating disabled people, and technologies are based on a view that a disability is a source of unhappiness for a person and humankind. To this, they make a counterargument, saying that a life with a disability is not necessarily unhappy, and prenatal testing should not be practised except for cases in which the test aims at saving the life of a foetus with anomalies (Sentensei shishi shōgaiji fubo no kai 1999; Yokota 2004).

Women's reproductive health movement groups contend that reproductive genetic technologies pressurise women to give birth only to healthy children, and therefore such technologies impede women's practice of their right to self-determination (Saitō 2002; Yokota & Yonezu 2004). They also maintain that reproductive genetic technologies should be practised under the condition there is no pressure on women to comply. There might also be women who want to give birth to a child knowing that the child has an anomaly, in such cases that one of the parents has a genetic disorder. In this case, they maintain that technology should be used to prepare the parents for safe delivery by the would-be mother, and to protect the life of the disabled child, but not to discriminate against the would-be children with anomalies. In short, both movements try to reaffirm the meaning of a disability, by denying the idea that a disability is a source of unhappiness for both individuals and society (Yokota & Yonezu 2004).

This sensitivity among the social movement groups about the value of a disability comes from the eugenic history of Japan. Japan has had laws on eugenics that stipulated legal sterilisation of disabled people in the name of 'preventing the birth of inferior offspring'.[2] Under the National Eugenic Law (1940-1948) and the Eugenic Protection Law (1948-1996), some 16,000 disabled women were sterilised, sometimes even without being notified.[3]

Medical associations are aware of this eugenic history in Japan, and are afraid of accusations from women's and disabled people's advocacy groups of being 'eugenic practitioners'. So, whenever they try to issue guidelines, they are careful in referring to a disability and selective abortion. For them, a disability is often a publicly untouchable issue (Kato 2007).

These are the main characteristics of public debates regarding the regulations of the practice of prenatal testing and selective abortion in contemporary Japan. There are quite a few scholarly analyses of the public debates regarding a disability, social movements, and the state regulations on prenatal testing (Ehara 1985; 1990; 1991; 1996; 1998; 2002; Ichinokawa 1996; Ichinokawa & Tateiwa 1998; Saito 2002).

A blind spot among scholarly analysis is, however, ordinary citizens' views on disabilities in the course of pregnancy. 'Ordinary citizen' is defined in a broader sense here. The majority of ordinary citizens are politically unallied with either the disabled people's movement or the women's reproductive health movement, and grew up having hardly anything to do with the issue of disabilities. They are without professional medical knowledge and never thought of what disabilities were till they became pregnant themselves, let alone considered the ethical or political meaning of pregnancy or risk in pregnancy. With hardly any medical knowledge, they suddenly appear before an obstetrician (OB hereafter) with anxieties as to whether the pregnancy will proceed smoothly and if the prospective child is healthy or not. Most visitors to OBs are actually citizens with these backgrounds. They are the ones deciding whether to test foetuses, and they are the practitioners of reproductive technologies in daily life. Yet, as far as this author knows, there is hardly any empirical research on the views of ordinary citizens on disability in Japan. This chapter aims to discuss the views on disabilities during pregnancy by ordinary citizens and how the views guide them in whether to undertake prenatal testing. Prenatal testing here includes maternal serum sampling (*kessei mākā tesuto*) and amniocentesis (*yōsui kensa*); chorionic villus sampling (*jūmō kensa*) is hardly practised and ultrasound (*chō-onpa*) is not considered to be a part of prenatal testing of pregnant women.

This chapter examines stories of six cases of pregnancy, collected during fieldwork in Japan (April to June 2006). In these cases, six women and four of their husbands were interviewed. All six come from Tokyo or its suburbs; none of the subjects has disabled people in their immediate family environments and grew up without paying special attention to disabilities; all were pregnant within the last three years; and none of them had any idea that they belonged to a high-risk group. This is important to note, because among pregnant women of advanced age, their age is often the direct link to higher-risk pregnancy. At the time of the interview, all of them expressed having had anxiety about the health of their foetus during pregnancy. Although sharing these similarities, three of the women underwent prenatal testing and three of them did not. This chapter intends to look at the decisive factors motivating individuals to take prenatal testing, paying attention to their views on disabilities.

Explanations about disability in Japan are also made in the light of previous empirical studies on decision-making regarding prenatal testing (Ozasa 2006; Sugano 2001; Tsuji 2003; Tsukamoto 2005), as well as other previous sociological, anthropological and folklore studies regarding health, abnormality, reproduction and family (Fujii 1993; Sugiyama-Lebra 1984; Takamune 1972; Takeda 1957; Yoshizumi 1995). The practice of ancestor worship (*senzo sūhai*) will be discussed mainly to focus on the cultural perspective of disability, reproduction and family lineage. In order to give a clearer explanation of what is observed among the six cases, this chapter also refers to the evidence from 46 other interviews, as well as specialists such as medical doctors and journalists who were interviewed at the same time as the six women. Out of 46 interviewees, 34 are women and 12 are their husbands. Details of the six interviewees are summarised in Table 7.1.

Approximately half of the 46 women were 'ordinary citizens' as defined here. Of the others, there are women with disabilities, those who experienced infertility treatment, and those who already had one disabled child or high-age pregnancy.

Anxiety about the health of the prospective child

First, this section looks at how pregnant women expressed their anxiety about the health of the prospective child. All the 46 pregnant women and their partners had some anxiety, which was not necessarily caused by either the presence of reproductive genetic technologies or their advancement. It was observed that wishes for a healthy child had been

Table 7.1 *Information on interviewees (Spring 2006)*

	Ms A (32)	Ms B (37)	Ms C (30)	Ms D (36)	Ms E (27)	Ms F (32)
Husband	Civil servant, 42. Interviewed.	Businessman, 37. Interviewed.	Computer programmer, 34. Not interviewed.	Businessman, 40. Interviewed.	Businessman, 40. Interviewed.	Physiotherapist, 31. Interviewed.
Family structure	Two children	First pregnancy	First pregnancy	Two children	First pregnancy	First pregnancy
Education	BA in Japanese literature	BA in music	MSc in computer science	High school	Junior college degree in designing	Junior college degree in nursing
Job	Fulltime housewife	Piano teacher	Computer programmer	Part time in supermarket	Part time self-owned business	Fulltime midwife
Religion	None	None	None	Buddhist	None	None
Prenatal testing	none	None	none	MSS	MSS, amniocentesis	MSS, amniocentesis

commonly shared by ordinary citizens regardless of whether one knew details about a disability, risk or prenatal testing. My field research shows that more than half of the 46 interviewees visit either temples or ancestors' graves to pray for the birth of a healthy child. Among the narratives, such statements were repeated as: 'Not to miss any bodyparts (*gotai manzoku*) is my only and greatest wish for the baby in my stomach'; 'It does not matter if it is intelligent or not, be beautiful or not, a boy or a girl. I only wish for the health for my child.' The health of a prospective child often becomes the primary concern of parents during pregnancy.

Yet, unless there is a certain genetic disorder in either the husband or wife's families, anxiety remains vague and unscientific. Although all the six main interviewees were trying to stay fit through exercise, or offering some kind of prayer, such as by visiting temples for a smooth pregnancy, hardly any were thinking of more technical tests than routine pregnancy procedures, such as urine tests and routine blood work. In terms of the sorts of disabilities that newborn babies might suffer, there was also scarce knowledge among pregnant women. The term *henna ko* (a weird child) was heard most frequently to refer to a child with an anomaly, in such statements as, 'What if this child in my stomach is *henna ko*?' (Ms A and C; Tsukamoto 2005: 124), yet, when asked what kind of anomalies they referred to, most of them could not provide either proper names of disorders or symptoms. Ms C, a computer programmer, stated that urine tests can detect autism with today's technologies, which is understood by her to be a chromosomal disorder, and Mr and Ms A could not tell the difference between Down's syndrome (DS) and cerebral palsy (CP).

Among the other 46 interviewees as well, those who had hardly had anything to do with disabilities in their lives knew little about disabilities or prenatal testing. The field research indicates that those who are disabled themselves and those who have family members with a disability know the most, accurately and technically, about prenatal testing and disabilities. Yet the tendency was also that even disabled people with non-genetic disorders, such as CP, were not interested in prenatal testing. All the interviewees with CP said: 'My disorder is not genetic, so I do not have to worry about this pregnancy so much (*idenbyō ja nai kara daijōbu*).'[4]

Overall, pregnant women are not sufficiently worried about an anomaly in a foetus as to seek information on prenatal testing. More 'gambling' attitudes are found towards reproduction. This does not mean that anxiety does not exist, nor, as will be discussed, that the fear of disability is naively unrecognised by pregnant women or their partners. Firstly, there are cultural values that transform anxiety into optimism in the course of pregnancy. Secondly, not knowing about a disability is also a means of maintaining their social identity, which is denied to disabled people. In other words, detailed knowledge about a disability or risk in pregnancy might make others think that one is anxious about being part of a risk group, and hiding that he or she has a genetic disorder. This point will be discussed later in this chapter.

The next section discusses the mechanism of cultural values that transforms anxiety into optimism during pregnancy.

Home-grown sense of statistics

While experiencing anxiety about the health of the prospective child, how do pregnant women manage to avoid thinking of having prenatal testing? This section discusses this point with a special focus on their view regarding disabilities.

Without my asking why, the following statements often naturally were offered to explain why they believed that the prospective child would not have a disability: 'because there are no relatives or family members with any disorders (*kazoku nimo shinsekinimo inai kara*)' (cases A, C, D and E); 'because the previous pregnancy experiences were also without problem' (Ms A and Ms D); 'my mother gave birth to me when she was older than my current age, so I am OK' (Ms C). Ms C continues:

> My mother gave birth to me when she was 38. The delivery was without problem. My elder sister gave birth to her first child when she was 33. I think our family line is strong (*uchi wa tsuyoi kakei nanda to omou*). I am 30, the youngest. I should not have any problem with my pregnancy. (translated by the author)

In this way, pregnant women tend to create certain images regarding the process, referring to previous pregnancies in their close families. This is called a 'home-grown sense of statistics', initially used by the US anthropologist Rayna Rapp (2000: 69). A home-grown sense of statistics is developed on the basis of one's own experience. Ms A, who gave birth to three children, describes her third pregnancy:

> Of course I would wonder whether the child was healthy or not. But the previous two pregnancies had been without problems – both were and still are healthy. I was experienced in giving birth, so I did not worry about the pregnancy. I did not think of taking any tests. (translated by the author)

In this way, experienced mothers develop greater conviction of the health of their babies. Rapp states, based on her research in New York, that a home-grown sense of statistics happens more frequently among those with low income, which actually implies their educational background and knowledge in reproductive genetics (2000: 68). In the context of perceptions of disability in Japanese society, based on this author's field research, hardly any significant correlation was found between education, income and genetic knowledge. On the contrary, pregnant women with a bachelor's degree as well as a master's degree (such as Ms C or Mr and Ms A) knew hardly anything about maternal serum sampling or amniocentesis. Among the other 46 interviewees, it was similarly found that almost half did not have precise knowledge about prenatal tests. For example, a junior high school teacher (33) with a bachelor's degree in pedagogy states, 'I read somewhere – I think it was in a maternal magazine – that if the first pregnancy turned out to be healthy by means of blood marker test, one does not have to take the test again during the next pregnancy. Because the test result means that you do not have sick genes.' The teacher did not recall the name of the magazine, and later she said that she probably had acquired this information from a friend, but she is not sure. Similarly, a university staff member (34) who holds a master's degree in psychology says, 'I saw that the department of ob-gyn was providing genetic consultations, but a genetic problem is relevant to those who have a certain disease. My pregnancy has nothing to do with genetic inheritance.' Reproduction, needless to say, has largely to do with genetic inheritance, if not a disorder. This account shows that genetic inheritance is equated with a matter of disorder by the interviewee. This explains how information is misunderstood and transmitted among ordinary citizens. The reason is primarily because genetics, including reproductive genetics, is not taught at school in Japan. Past history of eugenic practice in Japan means knowledge of genetics is equated with the ability to discern who is genetically inferior and superior.[5] Genetics is a taboo topic, including within the educational curriculum (Watanabe & Shimada 2005; Takebe 2002).

It should be noted that when pregnant women refer to other family members to explain their optimistic view about the health of the prospective child, they do this not only out of a mere sense of home-grown statistics, but also from conviction of a strong family lineage (often referred to as *uchi no kakei*). Recall the statement by Mr C: 'I think our family line is strong (*uchi wa tsuyoi kakei nanda to omou*).' Reference to their family line may connote common constitution and health pattern, but it was also possible to observe that the issue of the health of family line goes beyond a basic scientific account of physical and mental conditions. It also refers to cultural notions, such as the good fortune and protection that a family line enjoys. The next section explains the concepts of karma, or cause and effect, and family gods in the custom of ancestor worship (*senzo sūhai*).

Cultural concepts of family and disability

It was observed that pregnant women explained their optimism about the health of the prospective child saying, 'I am not worried because, as far as we know, there has never been the birth of an abnormal child either in my family or my husband's family' (Ms C), and 'Family lines of both my husband and mine do not have to do with disabilities' (Mr and Ms A). One might think that they refer to the genetic heritage of the family lines, but I want to focus on the meaning of these statements about family concerning the fact that more than half of the 46 interviewees – themselves and/or their family members – visit family graves and temples. This is in order to report their pregnancy to the ancestor and ask their ancestors to ensure the good health of the prospective child. At the same time, in case a disabled child is unexpectedly born in a family, such statements were heard from the interviewees as: 'my parents-in-law constantly ask themselves what kind of *in-nen* brought this sick child' or 'I was told by my parents-in-law that the birth of my child was *tatari* of my family line'. The terms *in-nen* and *tatari*, meaning 'direct and indirect causes' and 'punishment' respectively, are part of the custom of *senzo sūhai*, or ancestor worship. I will now look at the culture of ancestor worship and its link to the concept of health and disabilities.

In-nen is originally a Buddhism term based on the principle of karma, or cause and effect, which implies that 'because the ancestor of the family or I in the past life did something, may it be good or bad, the offspring of one's family receive the effect of it based on the principle of karma' (Takeda 1957: 216). The Japanese folklorist Fujii explains that, in Japan, there is an idea that a person who lived long and whose life ended naturally (*tenju o mattō suru*) becomes a god- or ghostlike figure (*hotoke, soshin*) of his/her family line (1993: 391). The ghost protects the family line, but sometimes metes out a kind of punishment (*tatari*) if the offspring does not properly pay attention to the ancestor, in the form of, for example, visiting the family grave (Fujii 1993). Some individuals implied that the birth of a disabled child was a sort of punishment, and others implied that the birth was a blessing using the concept of ancestor worship: *My daughter was born disabled to erase all the bad fortune of our family lines; we have to thank her.* Mr and Ms D, who lost their newborn child with Down's syndrome a few days after her birth, said that recovery of Mr D's father from cancer is because their child took the bad karma with her to another world.

The custom of visiting a family grave is also part of the rituals of *senzo sūhai* or worshipping ancestors. This is practised based on a household system as the basic unit, which is called *Ie*. *Ie* stands for family household, defined as a vertically composite form of nuclear families, one from each generation (Sugiyama-Lebra 1984: 20; 336). *Ie* is a line of inheriting family assets including surname, grave and property. The marriage system in Japan has, since the thirteenth century, taken the form of *yomedori kon*, or a woman entering the family line of her husband. In the system of *yomedori kon* in the context of the *Ie* household system, reproduction, especially producing a healthy boy as an heir, was seen to be the supreme mission of women. Traditionally, if a couple was infertile, the family of a husband was entitled to divorce her, calling the woman *umazume*, or a stone woman.

An interesting fact is that *Ie* continues successively not only from past to future through ancestors and descendants, but is also a conceptual and abstract family that continues even when family members all die off. Sometimes a *Ie* is resurrected by relatives, and it can exist even in the absence of actual family members and succeeding generations (Yoshizumi 1995: 186). Here, such intangible aspects as 'spirituality' and 'fortune', or *hotoke/soshin,* are important factors in assessing the quality of a *Ie* line. Quality refers not only to fertility, mental capacity and a healthy physical condition, but also towealth and social position. So, in the events of marriage and reproduction, the quality of a bride's family line was focused on not only fertility and health of offspring, but also whether the bride may bring good luck or bad luck to her husband's family line. This tradition is not as strong as it used to be, but still remains part of the cultural values in Japanese society, especially among parents-in-law and the parents' generation.

At the risk of becoming repetitive, it should be stressed that the line of the *Ie* household sharing the similar destiny is therefore different from genetic connection. It is sharing similar patterns in health, personality, constitution, good and bad fortune among members of the household and family lines, based on the same supernatural power or *kami*, gods. This can be explained by the fact that god- or ghostlike figures are shared by a *Ie* family line, where, since the emergence of the household system in the thirteenth century, adoption sometimes occurred to maintain one family line when there was no child in the family (Yoshizumi 1995: 186-187). When an adopted person entered a family line, the person was regarded to come under the common influence of the power of the same ancestors, sharing similar destiny and tendency in their lives, even if the person did not share what is now called genes. With regard to the cultural values of disability reproduction, it can now be concluded that people guess whether the prospective child has an anomaly or not, according to the health of the pregnant women and their partners in their family lines. They interpret the risk not only in genetic terms, but also in terms of the fortune of a family line. Furthermore, it can be said that the quality of offspring is interpreted to be an issue of luck in a family line, as the statements of Ms C as well as Mr and Ms A indicate.

This way of viewing life, based on ancestor worship, may not be the only way to interpret the birth of a disabled child, as, for example, pregnant women of advanced age associate risk first with their age, and those with disabilities think of risk in terms of medical knowledge. Terms such as *in-nen* and *tatari* are so much a part of daily vocabulary that individuals may not be quite aware what these concepts refer to. Yet these terms are worth discussing because they appear so often in conversations of ordinary people about the health of a foetus, and, by exploring the meaning of these terms, it is possible to understand the mindset of ordinary citizens regarding health and reproduction.

'I leave the health of my child to the will of *ten*'

The terms *kami* and *ten* were often heard in narratives as well. Pregnant women often state that 'there is no use in being worried so much about the health of my child (shinpai shitemo shikata ga nai). I leave everything to *ten* (*ten ni makaseru*)'. If the newborn child is disabled, parents, especially mothers, are first shocked to hear that their child is disabled, which might be followed by sadness and anger, but eventually almost all the mothers accept the fact, often transforming the event into something positive. In doing so, the following statement was heard from almost all the mothers who had a child with anomalies: '*Kami* gave me my child with an anomaly as a challenge for my growth as a person (*kami sama ga kureta chōsen*)'. *Kami* literally means god or gods, usually referring to a monotheistic god.

One would wonder what the term *kami* means in the context of these accounts, because the mothers also stated that they had no religion. The mothers who used this term were not Christian, Muslim or Hindu. As Japanese society is practically atheistic, most of its population has no specific religion that they put into practice on a daily basis. Seen from the fact that the term *kami* is juxtaposed to terms of *in-nen*, it is inferred that this concept, *kami*, is rather cultural, being understood in the context of ancestor worship as well. As the term *kami* is often heard when interviewees explain the event of pregnancy and the birth of disabled children, I want to go deeper into this concept to understand what the term means in the Japanese cultural context.

The Japanese folklorist Fujii Masao says, 'A deceased ancestor is in the view of gods (*kami*) in Japan' (1993: 391), and 'The concept of gods (*kami*) is synonymous with *ten*.' *Ten* literally means sky, but beyond the sky it means fate. It has to be noted that according to folklorist studies, the concept of *ten* and *kami* are both based on the custom of worshipping ancestors. *Kami* and *ten* are more abstract supernatural powers and fate beyond human's control.

In this way, it was possible to observe that people share a belief in something invisible, or a fate, which is different from a scientific logic, such as *in-nen*, *ten* and *kami*. So, when someone says, '*Kami* brought me this child with a disability', it means that a supernatural power, or fate, based on the ancestors' invisible influence on those living now, gave the child to the parents. With regard to how these terms are used, while the term *in-nen* tends to appear in the form of complaint about the birth of a child with an anomaly, *kami* is used in order to stay optimistic about the health of the prospective child. If the newborn child is disabled, the term is used in order to finally accept the fact; '*Kami* gave me this child to teach me about life.' Still, the birth of a disabled child is seen as negative, as the event needs reaffirmation with the help of the concept of *kami* or gods. *Kami* is good, but such pronouncements as, 'Because I was not living my life so seriously, *kami* gave me this child for me to learn more seriously about life,' were also heard. The term *ten* is also used to stay optimistic during pregnancy. *Ten* is an expression of a belief that there must be a protective force keeping the prospective child healthy.

Such terms are used not only by grandparents and in-laws, but also by young couples. Even if young couples are well acquainted with scientific knowledge, they at the same time refer to the family grave and deceased ancestors when talking about their anxiety about the health of the prospective child. Tradition, culture and scientific knowledge coexist around the event of reproduction. Though aware of the presence of risk and disorders in pregnancy, people resort to supernatural power, which is beyond cognitive conception, in order to feel at ease.

Tsukamoto, a Japanese scientist in nursing, also reports that the health of offspring is often translated in terms of prospective parents' moral deeds and the principle of 'cause and effect'. For example, one of her interviewees was told by her close friend that because she has been living her life so correctly with a sense of justice, without committing any wrong deeds (*kiyoku tadashiku ikitekita*), she does not have to be worried about the health of the prospective child. After hearing this from her friend, she could feel at ease during her pregnancy, because the pregnant woman believed that she had indeed been morally good in her life and therefore she could believe that her prospective child would be healthy (Tsukamoto 2005: 124). She continues to say, 'Had my way of living been unserious so far, I could have a chance to have a *weird child* (or *henna ko*)' (Tsukamoto 2005: 124).

Thus, it can be said that the health of the prospective child is interpreted based on the principle of cause and effect: not only that of ancestors and fortune of family members, but also one's own way of living. In other words, it can be interpreted that the birth of a disabled child is seen to be an effect of morally undesirable deeds. Although the terms are used positively, they are often juxtaposed with such expressions as 'it seems that I need more challenges in life' and 'I need to learn more seriously about life.'

Such are the accounts for the concept of disability expressed by those who do not know directly about disability. Unless one is familiar with the issue of disabilities, he or she does not go so far as to look for information about prenatal testing. Innocence prevails more widely among pregnant women and their partners during pregnancy. Yet some accounts indicate that not knowing about disabilities and prenatal testing can be a deliberate act to keep one's health identity, i.e. belonging to a group of non-disabled people and therefore not having to know about a disability or prenatal testing. The next section discusses this point.

Staying ignorant of prenatal testing is a deliberate act to maintain a social identity as non-disabled

So far, it has been observed that the conviction that the prospective child will be healthy comes from rather 'naive' attitudes towards pregnancy, in the sense that the conviction is based on misconceptions about pregnancy and unfamiliarity with disabilities. Yet another tendency was also found among interviewees, i.e. *not* thinking of risk as a deliberate act to make sure that one does not become affiliated with a disabled people's group. For example, to the question of how he thought about the health of prospective children, Mr A says:

> Pressure of discrimination toward disabilities exists in this society and I know that we might give birth to a disabled child. Having said that, I must say that I did not want to think about any unusual pregnancy tests, because I did not want to think of the possibility of having a disabled child in the family. To be honest, issues of disabilities are not our family's business (*shōjiki itte hitogoto*). Neither my family nor I belong to the discriminated; this is how I really feel it. When it comes to my family, there should be nothing wrong (*uchi wa daijōbu*). I believed that I did not have to know about any tests because we did not belong to a risk group. (translated by the author)

Expressing that for him, too, there is a possibility of having a child with a disability, Mr A said that he did not know about any means of prenatal diagnosis or screening, or about disorders that could be detected by reproductive genetic technologies. In fact, he explained that he had no opportunities to get to know about disabilities nor had he encountered any disabled people in his immediate environment.

Mr A is denying the possibility of having a disabled child without knowing about it. Two points can be raised here. It is possible to observe fear in his statement – 'fear' of what is unknown to him – and he is deliberately avoiding knowing what it is or thinking of the possibility of having a disabled child. It is often heard from among other interviewees with children with Down's syndrome that when they gave birth to a child with Down's syndrome, they did not know what it was and felt fearful about it, but as they came to know what it was, their fear decreased and they became able to confront the fact. In this way, a concept of unfamiliarity and an emotion of fear are often attached to a disability in Japan. Mr A knows that there is a chance of having a child with an anomaly, but in order to avoid feeling fearful, he deliberately avoided knowing what disabilities are, and what prenatal testing is.

The second point related to Mr A's statement is that, by not knowing about disabilities or prenatal testing, he tries to maintain his health identity and social identity. As he states himself, he thinks that thinking of the possibility of having a disabled child is what risk-group people do, and that, for him, not thinking of the possibility is a means to confirm that he and his family do not belong to a discriminated group. In other words, the fact he does not know about prenatal testing or disability is a victorious declaration that he belongs to a stronger group in society in terms of health and associations attached to health. Ms A, the wife of Mr A, further extends this identity to family identity. She states:

> The children of my younger sister and my husband's sisters are all healthy. It is taken for granted that my child is healthy, too. I do not have to worry that my pregnancy goes wrong. Moreover, my being worried would give unnecessary anxiety to my mother (*yokei na shinpai o kakeru*). Negative thoughts affect pregnancy in negative ways. I will give a healthy child to my parents as a piece of good family news. (translated by the author)

Previously, it was explained that individuals try to feel at ease about the health of the prospective child, looking at ancestors' and other family members' health. In the case of Mr and Ms A, it is observable that they are trying to prove that they are not exceptional in their family, in that all the newborn children are healthy. Cultural anthropologist Margaret

Lock's note is relevant here: 'In Japanese society the inability to perform one's role in a given group adequately generates a sense of not only having let oneself down, but of having let down the group as a whole' (Lock 1980: 248). In the context of Mr and Ms A, 'the inability to perform one's role' is compared to 'failure to give birth to a healthy child', the letting down of 'oneself' is compared to parents of the disabled child, and 'the group' is compared to 'the family lines'. Mr and Ms A are trying not to let down his family line, and his wife's, by breaking the sequence of having healthy children in his and his partner's family.

Thus, cultural perception of a disability in reproduction can be summarised as follows. Although anxiety is shared about the health of a prospective child, it is not always interpreted in terms of reproductive genetics. There is a prevailing atmosphere in society that one should not speak loudly about genetics, including reproductive genetics. Consequently, knowledge about genetics is not transmitted at schools either, and ordinary citizens hardly know about reproductive genetics. Similarly, disabled people, as well as issues of disabilities, are so isolated in society that non-disabled people do not even think of the possibility of having a disabled child in a realistic sense. Accordingly, unfamiliarity and fear grow around the issue of disability, and even to think of the possibility of having a disabled child could sometimes be stigmatised as 'what risk groups should do'.

This section has raised the issues of 'innocence' about a disability and 'deliberate avoidance' thinking regarding disability. Nevertheless, it has to be noted that these two characteristics coexist together in individuals, rather than there being one group of innocent people, and another who deliberately avoids thinking of a disability. One often does not know much about disabilities, being anxious and fearful at the same time.

So far, concepts of disabilities have been discussed focusing on cultural values prevailing in society. One might wonder in Japan, a society with such high technology and scientific development, how dissemination of scientific medical information happens and how this information leads citizens to decide whether to take prenatal testing. My field research data, as well as research by other scholars such as Tsukamoto (2005: 89), indicate that obstetricians are the greatest source of information about conditions during pregnancy, including prenatal testing: when pregnant women are anxious about the condition of their pregnancy, friends and family might give them advice from their experiences, but in the end, they ask their OBs for the final explanations of what is going on. Similarly, although increasing numbers of pregnant women nowadays obtain information through the Internet, they confirm the accuracy of the information with their OBs. It can be said, therefore, that OBs are the most trusted source of scientific and medical information for pregnant women. Then what attitudes do OBs have regarding dissemination of information on prenatal testing? The next section looks at OBs' attitudes and their interaction with ordinary citizens.

Attitudes of obstetricians in disseminating medical information

I interviewed eleven OBs during the same field research in which I interviewed 46 women on pregnancy: nine were amniocentesis specialists, one was an ultrasound specialist and one was a specialist in infertility treatments. All but one were specialists in prenatal diagnosis, who were able to talk about not only their own medical practice but the situation of prenatal testing in wider Japanese society. All revealed that they do not actively talk about prenatal testing on their own initiative; rather, they talk about the test methods when asked by patients. The following accounts discuss why they do not actively talk about prenatal testing (Kato 2007). When OBs refer to a test, it is understood by pregnant women to be a recommendation, and so OBs are usually careful not to casually mention tests and risks; most children are born healthy, so there is no need for taking a test; OBs' self-image is to give positive comments to clients about pregnancy and to relieve their anxiety. Talking about prenatal testing and risk in pregnancy are negative; OBs are afraid of being labelled eugenic practitioners by the disabled people's movement and women's movement as well as the mass media.

There is silence in Japan regarding the issue of reproductive genetics and, in general, regarding the issue of disability. Among OBs in Japan, there is a 'culture' to regard it more ethical not to mention the risk of having a foetus with an anomaly or reproductive genetic technologies to pregnant women. That OBs do not have to mention testing a foetus to pregnant women is declared even in state guidelines; the 1999 governmental guideline on maternal serum sampling (MSS) states that 'a medical doctor does not have to inform patients of prenatal test nor should the doctor recommend the test to clients'.[6] Also recently, both the Japanese Society of Obstetrics and Gynaecology and the Japanese Association of Obstetrics and Gynaecology together issued a guideline to the effect that 'OBs have no obligation (gimu) to inform that possibility of chromosomal disorder is estimated by means of ultrasound', because it leads to 'selection of life (inochi no senbetsu)' (Nishinihon shinbun, 31 March 2008).

In this selective silence, the field research data of this author indicates that 38 per cent knew or had heard of 'amniocentesis' and 6 per cent knew nothing about it at all (Kato 2007: 38). This number was contrary to expectation, as amniocentesis was introduced almost 40 years ago, and as MSS was a topic of much discussion regarding its ethical pros and cons after 1994 (Sugano 2001: 115).

Silence prevails. The intentions of the government, OBs and medical associations behind the series of regulations encouraging silence on prenatal screening are to prevent the routine practice of prenatal screening and selective abortion of disabled children. It can be said that the intention is meant to be ethical. Lacking sufficient information, who is then motivated to take prenatal testing and why? How do they experience taking the test? The next section looks at this point, focusing on the 'cultural concept of disability'.

Who chooses to have prenatal testing?

Now, I come back to the six cases to analyse what factors motivated three couples to undergo prenatal testing while the other three did not. Ms E and Ms F did MSS. Ms F opted for amniocentesis because of indications of a high likelihood of having a child with Down's syndrome (DS), while Ms E did not because the likelihood was low. Ms D had amniocentesis because ultrasound indicated the possibility of an anomaly in the foetus. To begin with, all six revealed that they did not know about the methods of prenatal testing, and initially none of the three considered taking prenatal testing. Not belonging to a risk group, they explained that they did not even imagine having a child with a disability (kangaemo shinakatta).

Then what drove the three couples to test the foetus? Ms E took the test because of her parents-in-laws' anxiety: a cousin on her husband's side of the family, and a nephew of her mother-in-law, has cerebral palsy (CP). CP is not a genetic disorder, yet, the parents-in-law wanted to make sure of the condition of Ms E's pregnancy. Ms E states:

> I do not want to bother myself with any test, but they constantly asked me how everything was going. I asked my OB for a test and heard that there is a blood test. That's easy. To be honest, I took the test only to set their mind at rest (anshin saseru tame). Otherwise, they would keep nagging me (shitsukoi). (translated by the author)

Interestingly, when asked about which disorders are detected by MSS, Ms E answered she did not know any. She continued that since she was a child, she had been told by her mother not to get close to disabled people, including those with Hansen's disease, and therefore she does not know about disabilities. Asked about what her mother meant, she answered she was not sure, but she guessed that her mother was worried that she would be attacked. Fear of the unknown, as well as a superior feeling due to not belonging to a disabled people's group, are found here. Ms E herself was not worried about her having a disabled child, and she took the test to make sure that the health of the prospective child was good.

Obviously, taking the test was not her intention. She does not know exactly what disabilities can be identified through MSS. Her main purpose is to calm down her parents-in-law. The Japanese genetic nurse Ozasa's analysis of pregnant women's decision-making about the test is useful here. She suggests that pregnant women decide to take a test based on a balance between the norms and expectations from her environment and her own desire (Ozasa 2006: 76-85). Norms and expectations are represented by family honour, and fear for disabled children expressed by other family members. Tsukamoto further explains that the less knowledge a pregnant woman has about prenatal testing and risk in pregnancy, the greater the chance that a pregnant woman is more influenced by the norm of her social surroundings (Tsukamoto 2005: 51).

As OBs are the most trusted source of information, their word can be a motive for individuals to take MSS, too. A couple's lack of knowledge and uncritical obedience to OBs may well cause confusion as well. The story of a couple (Ms and Ms F) is the best example of this:

> Ms F: My OB recommended that I take the Quattro test to make sure my pregnancy was in good condition. I thought, if a doctor says that, it must be worth checking. I did not expect anything bad. I completely believed that the test was to confirm that everything was going smoothly. But the result showed that it was more than 80 per cent likely that my child would have DS. Since then, my husband and I were in total confusion ... Then my OB mentioned amniocentesis, but I could not calmly think of it, because it then required us to think about abortion. But I took the test because my OB said so. The result of amniocentesis turned out to be negative. In retrospect, I did not understand what all those events were about.

> Mr F: Why did we have to suffer all this? I believed in what the doctor's said, that it was to make sure the pregnancy was going smoothly. But, in fact, I had so many sleepless nights ... During the next pregnancy, I will never take any of this kind of test again. Of course I will be worried about the condition of the pregnancy, but it will be a different kind of anxiety. I never want to experience this kind of suffering again.

Two points are observable here regarding why the couple took the test. First, the couple uncritically believed their OB's word. They thought the test must be necessary because their OB mentioned it. Similarly, to account for not having taken any prenatal test, Mr A explains: 'I did not think of any extra test because our OB did not mention anything about it. OBs are professionals in the field ... I thought that there would be no mistake if I only follow what medical doctors say.' Ms C also says: 'I do not have to think of any possibility of having a strange child (henna ko), because I believe my child is healthy. Why? Because my doctor says that it is healthy.'

In this way, an OB's reference to a test is an influential factor for individuals when considering prenatal testing. Second, it is also possible to observe casualness in the OB's words, i.e. 'the test is to hear good news'. This statement is probably based on the OB's clinical experience of most test results being negative; this is not only an incomplete truth, but even false information. OBs tend to talk positively about pregnancy, and it has to do with the OB's self-image mentioned earlier.

Among the 34 cases, six had MSS, eight had amniocentesis and one underwent CVS. For MSS, they cited the following issues (one interviewee named multiple reasons): to make sure that pregnancy is without problems (*anshin suru tame*, six); advanced age (five); already having one disabled child (one). With respect to amniocentesis, the following points were raised: ultrasound indicated a possibility of an anomaly in the foetus (five); MSS indicated high likelihood of having a child with DS (two); already having a disabled child (one). So, the main reasons for taking tests are advanced age and family history, including having a disabled child, as well as one of the parents having a chromosomal disorder. Sugano (2001: 115) and Tsukamoto (2005: 45) report the same result. In other words, risk-group people more realistically consider taking tests.

However, this chapter focuses on citizens who do not belong to a risk group. It can be concluded that among ordinary citizens, there is hardly any critical difference when it comes to the perception of a disability among ordinary citizens. All six shared an innocent idea about a disability and a more optimistic view about pregnancy. The factors that made a difference between those who took the test and those who did not were statements from OBs and pressure from their immediate social surroundings. Furthermore, they took the test in order to make sure that the pregnancy was going smoothly, hardly imagining they might have a disabled child. So, conviction that one would have a non-disabled child is more dominant than anxiety as a common factor among the six cases. It is noteworthy, though, that this innocence occasionally leads individuals to total confusion after being told of a high likelihood of having a child with DS, as seen in the case of Mr and Ms F.

Discussion

So far, it has been discussed that innocence and silence prevail around issues of disabilities and prenatal testing in Japan. Because of this innocence, ordinary citizens tend to believe that they have nothing to worry about concerning a disability in the course of a pregnancy. True, we probably do not have to be excessively obsessed by the health of the prospective child, so, in this sense, there is no major problem when pregnant women do not feel unnecessarily anxious about the pregnancy. Out of conscience, OBs do not talk about risk. They do not want to pressurise women into taking tests, nor do they want to discriminate against disabled people, as positive test results from prenatal testing often lead to termination, which is viewed to be ethical. It was also observed that even the governmental guidelines tend to stay silent about disability or prenatal testing. Educational curricula contain hardly any genetic subject matter during high school, or even at medical schools, because it is a taboo topic. Silence forms the foundation of the ethics of prenatal testing and disabilities in Japan.

Yet, we have seen that the silence is producing 'fear' of the unknown among ordinary citizens, which sometimes creates a stigma on the birth of a disabled child ('you or your ancestor did something and therefore, the newborn child is disabled'). Pressure weighs on both parents, and yet, traditionally, the quality of women's health or women's family line's health has been named the cause of a problem, but it can be said that this stigmatisation is, by and large, illegitimate oppression of women whose children are born with an anomaly (Tsuji 2003: 49-50). At any rate, there is always a possibility of having a disabled child.

Now, the question is, to what extent can we manage to hide a disability and a function of prenatal testing from ordinary citizens by being silent? Is a lack of information about a disability or the means of testing a foetus true protection for the ordinary citizens in the long run? On the contrary, if we inform patients about disability, can we not expect that prenatal testing will reduce cultural taboos around living with a disability? At any rate, it seems to be impossible to keep hiding information on disabilities, risk, pregnancy and prenatal testing. The Internet is so accessible that ordinary citizens easily obtain information about prenatal testing. The average age of women giving birth is increasing, so the anxiety about risk in pregnancy will soon become a common issue in Japan. Furthermore, the reality is that an increasing number of disorders are able to be discovered by means of prenatal testing. The government and medical associations tend to employ silence in their guidelines, believing that to be an ethic protecting both medical doctors and patients. I conclude this chapter by saying that what is considered to be ethical, in this case 'silence', in Japan might actually not be ethical but might function to endanger the knowledge of ordinary citizens in the long run. This question needs discussion involving various levels of citizens. In my view, to employ the concept of creating 'wise patients' (Arimori 2005: 117-122), in order to prevent such cases as Mr and Ms F, would make for 'good governance' on prenatal testing in Japan.

Notes

1 There is no official figure on selective abortion, but according to the interviews with obstetricians, more than 90 per cent of positive test results lead to termination of pregnancy.
2 The first sentence of the Eugenic Protection Law.
3 The Asahi Shimbun. 14 February 1996. Yûseihogohôkaisei tachiba no sa. Tokyo.
4 This statement was heard even from among those with CP actively involved in disabled people's movement against reproductive genetic technologies and selective abortion. It was possible to observe that they were also caught in a dilemma, between personal hope for a healthy child and political belief against prenatal screening.
5 For example, it has been a tradition for business companies to investigate the health of all members of the family of the candidate as a procedure of selection. In particular, it is investigated whether there have been any hereditary, mental, or other debilitating diseases among the relatives of the applicants. This investigation is called *katei chôsa*. Knowledge in genetics has been used in this way, namely to select people without genetic problems (Rohlen 1974: 71).
6 The Ministry of Health and Welfare, www1.mhlw.go.jp/houdou/1107/h0721-1_18.html

8   Genetic Tests and Insurance in Japan: The Case for a Regulatory Framework

Gerard Porter

Introduction

In contrast to the position in many advanced industrial countries, Japan lacks a specific regulatory framework to govern the ways in which insurance companies can make use of genetic test results. Whilst this situation has not yet given rise to major social or legal problems, this article nevertheless argues that the current policy vacuum is unsatisfactory. Some options for the development of an appropriate regulatory system are suggested, drawing from the recent experiences of countries such as Australia and the United Kingdom, whilst taking into account some particular features of the Japanese insurance market.

Genetic tests can be used to predict an individual's risk of developing particular diseases. This can enable improved medical care and also help inform reproductive decisions (Godard et al 2003). Proposals to make use of genetic test results outside the healthcare context in areas such as insurance underwriting, however, have proved highly controversial (Markman 2004; Miyachi 2004).

Three main arguments have been raised against the use of genetic test results by insurers. First, people fear that allowing insurers to use genetic tests would lead to the emergence of a socially and economically marginalised 'genetic underclass'. Second, it has been argued that treating people less favourably on the basis of genetic characteristics constitutes an unacceptable form of 'genetic discrimination'. Third, some evidence suggests that individuals may be deterred from undergoing genetic tests due to concerns that an adverse result could disqualify them from the insurance market. For diseases where effective medical interventions exist, the disincentive to take clinically valuable tests could potentially lead to an increase in otherwise preventable deaths (Armstrong et al 2003).

Those arguing in favour of allowing insurers to make use of genetic test results, meanwhile, emphasise the fact that insurance is a private arrangement that operates according to the principles of freedom of contract and free market competition (Ashcroft 2007). Insurers conducting business in this environment have a legitimate commercial interest in using genetic tests to differentiate between high- and low-risk applicants, and to then assign individuals to the categories that most accurately reflect the degree of risk they carry (Holm 2007). Insurance companies have long used predictive information, such as medical history and family history, to assess and select risk, and argue that using genetic information in this way would simply be a logical extension of current practice (Miyachi 2004; O'Neill 1998; Tarr 2002). Indeed, allowing insurers to make use of genetic test results may actually help some people to obtain insurance, as a test result revealing that an individual is free from a particular genetic mutation can be used to cancel out negative inferences that might otherwise be drawn from family history (Tarr 2002).

It has also been asserted that insurers would be vulnerable to financial losses through 'adverse selection' (Akerlof 1970; Siegelman 2004) if they were prohibited from requesting the results of genetic tests. Adverse selection could occur if people who had undergone a genetic test, and knew that they had a high risk of falling ill or dying within the insured period, concealed this information from insurers and took out policies with the highest possible payouts (Ashcroft 2007). The losses sustained due to asymmetries of information and mispricing of risk would be unfair to individual companies and also to other policy holders, who would likely be forced to pay higher premiums to cross-subsidise high-risk individuals. Some scholars have suggested that if adverse selection were to occur on a major scale, it could lead to a 'death spiral' (Siegelman 2004) that would threaten the collapse of the insurance industry (Miyachi 2000).

The debate over whether insurers should have access to genetic test results has been notably difficult to resolve, with the various points of contention often reflecting broader underlying disagreements about the nature, social function and limits of private insurance in modern societies. Despite these complexities, many countries have constructed regulatory frameworks which aim to clarify the ways in which and the extent to which insurers are able to make use of genetic tests results and genetic information. National approaches have varied greatly in form (e.g. legislation, moratoria and industry self-regulation) and in substance (i.e. from highly restrictive to permissive approaches) (Godard et al 2003; Lemmens et al 2004; McGleenan 2000).

In the United States, for example, the Genetic Information Non-discrimination Act (GINA), signed into federal law in May 2008, makes it unlawful for health insurers to deny coverage or charge a higher rate or premium to otherwise healthy individuals on the basis of their genetic information.[1] Insurance companies in Austria, Belgium, Denmark, Estonia, France, Luxembourg and Norway are also prohibited from asking applicants to undergo genetic tests or disclose genetic test results (Godard et al 2003; Halldenius 2007). The Netherlands, Sweden and the UK, meanwhile, have adopted a 'ceiling approach', whereby insurers can only make use of genetic test results for certain kinds of policies above a certain threshold value. Industry guidelines in Australia are more permissive, and allow the use of genetic test results, but establish obligations on insurers to explain their reasons for adjusting premiums or policy conditions, and also to take account of the benefits of special medical monitoring and early medical treatment when assessing overall risk (IFSA 2005).

By comparison, the regulatory response in Japan has been somewhat ambivalent. A commitment to the prohibition of 'genetic discrimination' has been expressed in two sets of guidelines: the Fundamental Principles of Research on the Human Genome, issued by the Council for Science and Technology Bioethics Committee in June 2000, and the Guidelines for Genetic Testing, produced by the Genetic-Medicine-Related Societies in August 2003. These guidelines, however, are of little real impact due to their piecemeal and non-binding nature. The Japanese government does not appear to have plans to introduce more concrete safeguards in the foreseeable future. The insurance industry's position is also unclear, as no explanations have been given as to how insurers intend to assimilate genetic testing within their actuarial practices (Achim 2004). This silence may well signify that Japanese insurers have yet to formulate a coherent policy.

In the absence of a concrete framework, the use of genetic information by insurers is governed by the general provisions regulating insurance contracts found within the Japanese Commercial Code. The first legal dispute in this area was heard by the Osaka High Court in 2004. This ruling (discussed below) went some way to clarifying how the general principles of Japanese insurance law will be applied to genetic test results, but ultimately left several important policy questions unanswered. To some Japanese academics, medical societies and a proportion of the Japanese public, the current policy vacuum is cause for concern (Macer & Chen Ng 2000; Okada 2001). This paper critically analyses the issues raised and offers suggestions for reform.

The paper is divided into five parts. Part I highlights what is at stake in the debate by explaining why access to private insurance in Japan matters. Part II discusses the incidence of 'genetic disease' in Japan, whilst Part III outlines the current legal framework regulating the use of genetic information and genetic test results by Japanese insurers, and also discusses the implications of the aforementioned 2004 Osaka High Court ruling. Part IV argues that whilst the incorporation of scientifically validated genetic test results into underwriting practices – as has been the approach in Australia – would not constitute 'discrimination', it may still have adverse social consequences if it were to deter people from undergoing testing. With this argument in mind, Part V concludes the paper by offering suggestions for the development of a regulatory framework in Japan, drawing upon the approach in the UK and taking into account some particular features of the Japanese private insurance market.

Part I: Public and private insurance in Japan

One of the major concerns raised by the advent of genetic testing in Japan is access to insurance (Miyachi 2005). Although the Japanese public health insurance system provides universal coverage for most healthcare costs (NIPSSR 2007), being denied private health insurance coverage may still have adverse economic consequences for individuals and their families. Citizens insured under employer-based insurance schemes or the National Health Insurance system pay a modest monthly premium which entitles them to a 70-90 per cent reduction in their medical bills (Ramseyer 2007). Co-payments under the employer-based schemes and the National Health Insurance are currently capped at 140,000 yen[2] (approximately US $ 1,300) per month, plus 1 per cent of the excess over a certain sum (Ramseyer 2007). These arrangements have, however, been placed under increased financial pressure due to the costs of providing medical care to the growing elderly population in Japan. Recent rises in out-of-pocket expenses have increased patients' financial burdens, and instilled a sense of anxiety amongst the Japanese public about the future of the public health insurance system (Japan Center for Economic Research 2005). It is against this backdrop that the Japanese private medical insurance market has seen substantial growth in recent years (JETRO 2005; Suzuki 2005).

According to figures issued by the Japanese Ministry of Health, Labour and Welfare (MHLW), 57.9 per cent of Japanese people aged over 18 and over 70 per cent of people in their 30s and 40s have taken out private health insurance (Suzuki 2005). Policies typically pay a fixed benefit each day a person is hospitalised or undergoes one of the surgical procedures listed within the policy (Japan Center for Economic Research 2005). Insurers have also developed cheaper policies that provide coverage for a limited range of specified diseases. Cancer insurance has been a particularly successful example of this kind of specialised product (JETRO 2005). Although private health insurance fulfils an income protection function, most Japanese view these products as representing a means to offset the rising burden of treatment and other associated costs (Imanaka et al 2004; Suzuki 2005). The number of long-term nursing care insurance policies purchased in Japan is also increasing steadily, though it is still lower than the number of private medical insurance policies.

Access to private life insurance is also an important policy issue. The Japanese life insurance market is well established, and according to a survey conducted by the Japanese Institute of Life Insurance (JILI) in 2003, 89.6 per cent of all Japanese households have at least one life insurance policy attached to a family member (JETRO 2005). In cases where life insurers reject high-risk applicants on the basis of adverse genetic test results (rather than simply loading premiums), individuals will be unable to make provisions for the financial security of their dependants after their death, a situation that could cause serious economic hardship in certain cases.

Other additional factors must also be considered. The infrastructure enabling the use of genetic testing in the clinical context has only been established in Japan fairly recently, but it has been suggested that the use of genetic tests for healthcare purposes may gradually become more commonplace in the coming years (Matsuda 2003). Troublingly, this medical technology is being introduced into a society where families with members suffering from hereditary conditions have often been stigmatised. The particular fear that marriage prospects will be reduced for all family members (Kneller 2001) has lead to a cultural tendency (especially in rural areas) to keep the existence of genetic conditions a closely guarded family secret (Macer 2003). Commentary suggests that even in contemporary Japan, genetic disease remains a 'taboo' subject for many Japanese (Mutō 2000; Stuart 2000).

In light of the ongoing transitions in clinical practice in Japan, the demographic challenges facing the Japanese welfare state, the cultural sensitivities surrounding genetic disease and the current lack of legal clarity, it would be advisable for stakeholders to begin to consider some of the issues raised by genetic testing and their potential ramifications for Japanese insurers and insurance applicants (Achim 2004).

Part II: Genetics and disease in Japan

Comparative population studies indicate both similarities and differences between Japan and other countries in relation to the prevalence of genetic disorders. Although the frequency of conditions such as Duchenne muscular dystrophy, haemophilia A and chromosomal abnormalities in Japan is around the same as that found amongst Caucasian populations (Matsuda 2004), for many of the serious, late-onset genetic conditions of more relevance to insurance companies (Greely 2001; Mittra 2007; O'Neil 1998), the percentage of people affected in Japan is significantly less (Miyachi 2005).

Huntington's disease, for example, is a rare condition in the UK, with a prevalence rate of 4-10 per 100,000 individuals. The condition is rarer still in Japan, with a prevalence rate of just 0.5-0.6 per 100,000. In 1998, the total number of registered Huntington's patients in Japan was 526, compared to the far higher figure of around 5000 individuals in the UK (Mutō 2000: 17). Breast cancer affects 1 in 8 women in the United States but only 1 in 40 women in Japan, although it is estimated that around 60 per cent of familial breast and ovarian cancers in Japan involve the BRCA1/2 mutations (Arai et al 2004; USNIH 2006).

By contrast, rates of colorectal cancer have risen rapidly in post-war Japan to reach levels comparable with that of the US. Surprisingly, Japanese migrants to the United States have higher rates of colorectal cancer than the host population (Flood et al 2000; Marchand 1999). Ongoing epidemiological studies suggest that certain genetic characteristics found within the Japanese population, such as the NAT2 and CYP1A genetic mutations, in conjunction with eating a diet high in red meat, may increase susceptibility to colorectal cancer.

This brief comparative overview suggests that even taking into account the relatively high rates of colorectal cancer in Japan, it is probable that only a small section of the Japanese population would potentially be disadvantaged by the integration of genetic test results into insurance underwriting practices. The following section will discuss the manner in which this subgroup may be affected by outlining the current legal and regulatory framework in Japan pertaining to the use of genetic information by insurers.

Part III: The regulatory framework for genetic tests and insurance in Japan

A: Principles of private insurance under the Japanese Commercial Code

Insurance systems such as the Japanese public health insurance system and the UK's National Health Service operate under the principle of 'solidarity'. Participation is compulsory and coverage is universal, regardless of risk status or ability to pay (Mittra 2007). Private insurance schemes, by contrast, operate under the principle of 'mutuality' (Murata 2001). This means that purchase is optional and only by mutual agreement between the insurer and the applicant, in accordance with the principles of freedom of contract and free market competition (Wilkie 1997). Prospective customers are therefore free to purchase the most competitive insurance policies for their particular needs, whilst insurers can either undertake or reject individual applicants on the basis of their health status or other factors, and can also set the prices of their insurance premiums in accordance with the degree of risk that each particular applicant carries. This industry practice is known as 'risk selection' (Miyachi 2004).

The legal framework established by the Japanese Commercial Code is supportive of the principles of mutuality and freedom of contract that underpin private insurance markets. Articles 644 and 678 of the Code facilitate the process of risk selection by placing insurance applicants under a duty to disclose all facts relevant to their application ('the duty to disclose') (Okada 2001). The same articles also make it clear that insurers may rescind an insurance contract in cases where the insured party did not disclose important matters or made untrue reports concerning material facts at the time of making the contract due to bad faith or gross negligence (Ishihara 2002).

Japanese life and health insurance application forms require applicants to disclose information concerning their personal medical history and lifestyle in order to allow insurers to assess the likelihood of a claim being made during the term of the policy (Miyachi 2005; Murata 2001; Otomo 2005). One unusual – and highly significant – feature of Japanese practice is that insurance application forms do not generally require details relating to family history of disease (Miyachi 2005: 112). This contrasts with the position in countries such as the UK, where family history is routinely requested and used for risk selection purposes because of its value in indicating the presence or absence of hereditary conditions (Morrison 2005). Miyachi observes that although Japanese insurance forms did at one time request family medical history (i.e. details concerning the applicant's parents, children and spouse), from 1974 onwards the industry developed a policy of 'self restraint' and stopped asking for this information (2005: 112). This self-imposed restriction may well be re-examined in light of the current debate on the appropriateness of the use of genetic tests in insurance underwriting (Miyachi 2005: 112). Apart from this striking anomaly, methods of risk selection in Japan are generally in line with standard international practice. For example, insurance companies in Japan may sometimes request that applicants undergo a supplementary medical examination in order to get a clearer idea of current and likely future health status (Miyachi 2005: 115).

Applicants found to be in good health will usually be charged at ordinary rates, whereas those in poor health or with higher health risks will likely be assigned to higher risk bands and charged higher premiums. In extreme cases where an applicant's health risk is so high as to make insurance a commercially non-viable option, the insurer may decline coverage altogether. The industry practice of only selecting applicants carrying low to moderate risks whilst rejecting high-risk applicants is known as 'cream skimming' or 'cherry-picking' (Mittra 2007; Miyachi 2005). It is important to recognise that in Japan, as elsewhere,

risk selection practices based on medical data can mean that some individuals are excluded from the market. Thus, despite the socio-economic
importance of private insurance in contemporary Japan, there is no legal 'right' as such to life insurance or private health insurance.

B: Non-binding guidelines relating to genetic testing and insurance

Two sets of Japanese guidelines express a normative commitment to
prohibiting what is referred to as 'genetic discrimination' in the context
of insurance. The first of these is found in the Fundamental Principles
of Research on the Human Genome (the Fundamental Principles),
which is a set of research guidelines issued by the Bioethics Committee
of the Council for Science and Technology (a Cabinet Office policy
council comprising the Prime Minister, relevant ministers and expert
advisors) in June 2000. The Fundamental Principles bear a degree of
resemblance to the 1997 UNESCO Universal Declaration on the Human Genome and Human Rights in their tone and approach. Principle
16 ('Prohibition of discrimination') of the Fundamental Principles states
that:

> The genetic information of a participant forms the basis of his/
> her diversity as a member of humanity. The participant should
> not be subjected to any discrimination on account of any genetic
> characteristic in his/her genetic information that is obtained
> from the research.

The explanatory note to this provision mentions insurance as one area
where 'discrimination' may occur. However, the provision neither defines the term 'discrimination' nor clarifies how genetic information
should be handled in contexts other than genomic research, e.g. clinical
practice. Furthermore, as the Fundamental Principles are not legally
binding, this provision is of limited practical effect.

The second example of an attempt to protect the interests of those
undergoing genetic tests can be seen in the Guidelines for Genetic Testing (the Guidelines) (2003), which is a set of ethical principles issued
by the Genetic-Medicine-Related Societies – a group of ten medical organisations involved in the provision of genetic testing services in Japan. Section 2.2 of the Guidelines provides that '[a]ll efforts should be
made to protect examinees and/or relatives from possible discrimination (genetic discrimination) on the basis of their genetic information'.
Furthermore, Section 3.2 states that:

> Individual genetic information gained from testing must be sub-
> ject to confidentiality, and therefore fundamentally should never

be disclosed to relatives or any third party without obtaining permission from the examinees themselves. Even when the examinees agree, individual genetic test results should be protected from access by employers, health insurers and schools.

This surprising provision establishes an obligation on members of the Genetic-Medicine-Related Societies to withhold genetic test results from insurers, even if authorised to forward this information by the individual concerned. The provision is, however, of questionable practical effect, as it does not change the fact that an insurance applicant has a legal duty to disclose all material information when applying for insurance, including the fact of having taken a genetic test (although in some cases it may make it more difficult for insurers to access relevant medical records to prove that insured parties have breached this duty). The Guidelines are concerned solely with the interests of examinees, and do not engage with the question of how any adverse selection that might arise would affect insurers' interests. At the current time, there is little concrete information available describing how this particular provision has been applied in practice. It is interesting to note that neither of these two sets of guidelines was mentioned in the 2004 insurance case discussed below.

In the absence of any clear regulatory framework, the use of genetic information is governed, by default, under the standard principles for the regulation of insurance contracts contained within the Japanese Commercial Code. At the current time, Japanese insurance companies are not making systematic use of genetic test results; they do not require applicants to undergo tests as a condition of their application, and it is considered highly unlikely that there will be any shift from this policy in the future (Miyachi 2005). However, it is also generally thought by Japanese scholars that if an applicant has already undergone a genetic test, then the result of this test would be considered as information material to the insurance contract for the purposes of risk selection and would therefore fall within the scope of information to be disclosed by the applicant under the provisions of the Commercial Code (Ishihara 2002).

The first example of civil litigation in the area of genetic testing and insurance has already been decided by the Japanese courts. This ruling goes some way toward clarifying how the Commercial Code will be applied to govern the use of genetic test results by Japanese insurers, but adopts a particularly strict view of knowledge and disclosure with potentially far-reaching consequences in the realm of genetics.

C: The 2004 Osaka High Court 'Insurance Money Request' Case

We might expect most instances of disputes over the use of genetic test results by insurers to occur at the stage when a high-risk applicant initially tries to take out an insurance policy. However, this first Japanese test case did not centre upon a pre-contractual dispute involving an asymptomatic individual being refused insurance coverage because of an adverse predictive test result. Rather, the case was a post-contractual dispute over the issue of whether an insurance company could avoid its obligation to pay a sum specified under an insurance contract, because a later diagnostic test revealed that the insured party was suffering from a genetic disorder at the time of entering into the contract. This situation occurred because of some particular features of the standard terms in which Japanese health insurance contracts are set out.

The ruling of the court of first instance, the Kobe District Court,[3] was issued in 2003, and the appeal ruling by the Osaka High Court was made the following year, in 2004.[4] This is the first case of its kind in Japan, but with the possibility of the clinical use of genetic tests becoming more commonplace in the coming years, may well be the first of many.

The plaintiff (X) entered into a combined life, health and severe disability insurance contract with *Dai-Ichi Seimei Hoken Sogo Kaisha*, a large and well-known firm of insurers in Japan. Article 1 of the policy stipulated that the payment of money in the event of 'severe disability' under the insurance contract would be restricted to the following circumstances:

> ... severe disability occurring during the period of liability on the part of the insurers that is caused by injury or illness that arises *after* the period of the commencement of liability. This includes cases where pre-existing injuries or medical conditions have no causal relationship with the severe disability occurring after the commencement of liability on the part of the insurer [emphasis added]. (Yamashita 2004)

This kind of exclusion clause is a standard term within Japanese health insurance contracts, and one which supports the ability of insurance companies to select risk and avoid losses that may occur due to adverse selection (Hasegawa 2005).

Since he was a primary school child in 1973, X had had difficulty walking. He received muscle-tissue transplants in both legs in 1975 and 1976. The transplants improved his condition, and X progressed to high school and university, but from the period from 1979 to 1985 he still consulted with a specialist once a year to monitor his condition. X graduated from university and entered into employment. After being approached by a sales representative from the *Dai-Ichi Seimei* insurance company, X decided to purchase a combined life and health insurance policy, which contained a clause for the payment of medical treatment for 'severe disability'.

Under the policy, X would be able to claim 5000 Japanese yen (approximately US $ 46) per day for medical expenses relating to the treatment of 'severe disability' as defined within Article 1 of the contract, as well as a full and final lump-sum payment of 10,000,000 Japanese yen (approximately US $ 93,000) for 'severe disability' – again, as defined within Article 1. The severe disability insurance policy would terminate upon payment of the final lump sum.

X satisfied the legal duty to disclose all known facts material to the application, and gave full details of his medical condition at that time, as well as of all the medical treatment that he had received up until that point. Following a separate medical examination by a doctor representing the insurance company, X was then allowed to enter the insurance scheme. Contractual relations commenced from 12 October 1989. In 1990, however, X's condition suddenly deteriorated to the point that he was no longer able to walk, and he was classified as being a physically handicapped person in 1992. Soon after X had been classified as disabled, he approached the insurance company with the intention of making a claim under the insurance contract. The branch office manager assured X that he would receive the money under the severe disability policy, but recommended that because the policy would terminate once the final lump sum had been paid, it would be in X's best interests to continue paying the insurance premiums so that he could also claim back expenses for any future medical treatment relating to his severe disability. X could then make an application for the lump-sum payment at a later date following the completion of his medical treatment. X acted in accordance with this advice.

X decided to undergo a further series of medical tests in order to establish the cause of his condition. In March 1994, due to the low levels of the enzyme galactosylceramide beta-galactosidase indicated by his blood test, X was diagnosed as having late-onset Krabbe disease – a rare inherited disorder of the nervous system (National Institute of Neurological Disorders and Stroke, 2008). There have been few documented cases of this disease in Japan.

X put in a claim for the final lump-sum payment of 10,000,000 Japanese yen with his insurance company in 1999. However, after having reviewed X's claim application, the company informed him that, in accordance with the aforementioned stipulation regarding the condition of payments for severe disability, his application had been rejected. The company stated that the genetic test result of March 1994 had indicated

that X was already suffering from Krabbe disease well before the commencement of contractual liability, and that his pre-existing medical
condition had simply worsened during the insured period. The company asserted that under Article 1 of the insurance contract, claims for
severe disability where the illness had begun before the commencement of the contract would be excluded.

X sued for payment of the lump sum under the insurance contract.
The court of first instance, the Kobe District Court, rejected the plaintiff's arguments and found in favour of the insurance company. The
Court's reasoning was centred on adopting a strict, literal interpretation
of the aforementioned contractual provision, and upon applying an objective, scientific approach to assess the precise timing of the onset of
X's illness, which it stated was in 1973 when X was a schoolchild and
first began to have difficulties walking. X appealed to the Osaka High
Court.

D: Summary of the 2004 Osaka High Court Ruling

X's appeal was successful. The Osaka High Court ordered the insurance
company to pay X the requested lump sum of 10,000,000 Japanese
yen. Although most of the substantive points in the ruling went against
X, as the Osaka High Court approved the Kobe District Court's approach to the objective assessment of the aforementioned contractual
provision and the timing of the onset of the disease, the Osaka High
Court nevertheless found for X on the grounds that the insurance company had breached its duty to act in good faith. The court observed that
when X had been diagnosed as being disabled in 1992, and had approached the insurance company with regards to making a claim under
the severe disability insurance contract, the branch office manager had
informed X that he would be awarded payment under the severe disability policy. Upon consideration of the scope of the insurance company's operational responsibilities towards its customers, as well as the
greater degree of knowledge possessed by the company representatives,
the Osaka High Court found that the company's subsequent decision to
renege on this statement constituted a breach of good-faith requirements.

Although the ruling therefore ultimately hinged on a fairly narrow
technical issue, the case is nonetheless important for the broader precedent it sets. The following section looks at three points to emerge from
this judgement that will be of relevance in instances where insurers do
not breach the duty to act in good faith by retracting earlier statements
that payouts will be made.

E: Broader implications of the 2004 Osaka High Court ruling

i: Retrospective application of exclusion clauses

The first legal point to be clarified by the ruling is that if an insured party was manifesting symptoms of a disease (such as a genetic disorder) at the time of entering into a standard insurance contract, insurers will not be obliged to make payouts in relation to claims arising from the worsening of that pre-existing medical condition. This rule applies even in cases where the insured party has acted in good faith by disclosing to the best of their knowledge all relevant information relating to their personal medical history at the time of entering into the contract, and even in cases where the medical technology for diagnosing the particular medical condition was not available at the time the contract was formed.

On one level, the approach adopted by the Osaka High Court on this point is understandable, as it is consistent with previous Japanese rulings where exclusion clauses for 'pre-existing medical conditions' have been interpreted in a broad, expansive fashion (Amari 2006). An illustrative example can be provided by a 1990 ruling by the Supreme Court of Japan.[5] Here, an exclusion clause was interpreted in a case where an insured party, who suffered from nerve damage in both eyes, was left blind after being involved in a traffic accident which occurred after the commencement of the contract. The Supreme Court held that the insurer was not obliged to pay the benefits stipulated under the policy because the plaintiff's pre-existing optical nerve damage was viewed as one cause of the disability that arose during the insured period. To foreign legal scholars, this approach is likely to seem unduly harsh.

The policy rationale generally offered by the Japanese courts has been that such an approach is necessary to maintain the 'predicted accident occurrence rates' that form the statistical basis for insurance underwriting (Amari 2006). This argument is unpersuasive. It is well known that in reality, risk pools, constructed with reference to actuarial tables, are not populated by homogeneous groups of individuals who each bear identical levels of insurance risk. Even in situations where risk selection mechanisms function correctly and applicants are truthful in their pre-contractual disclosure of material facts, a few individuals who are unaware of their own high-risk status will inevitably slip through the net and end up being allocated to risk pools that result in them paying a lower premium than is appropriate for their actual level of risk. But over time, in the absence of adverse selection problems, results should average out for an appropriately constructed risk pool (Tarr 2002).

Given this fact, it is far from clear that the economic losses faced by insurers would be of a magnitude that justifies the exclusion of insurers' liability in the small number of cases with fact patterns similar to the 2004 Osaka High Court case. It is also worth noting that Japanese courts have not produced any empirical evidence to support their assertion that it is essential to shield insurers from liability in marginal cases where no adverse selection (Akerlof 1970; Siegelman 2004) has occurred.

In addition, the Japanese judiciary's failure to draw any ethical distinction between prospective and retrospective cherry-picking by insurance companies in cases where the applicant has acted in good faith raises fundamental issues of fairness in contractual interpretation. When faced with similar scenarios, Anglo-Commonwealth courts have focused on the question of whether or not the insured party satisfied the duty to act in utmost good faith by disclosing all relevant facts to the insurer at the time of making the application. When applying this doctrine, courts have refused to penalise individuals for failing to disclose pre-existing risks manifesting after the commencement of contractual relations, but which the insured party could not have reasonably known about when entering into the contract.[6] The Anglo-Commonwealth approach thus acknowledges the importance of maintaining industry profitability, but ultimately views commercial interests as representing just one set of concerns that must be balanced within a matrix of competing factors (which include the gravity of the consequences of transferring the loss to one or the other party, the moral significance of acting in good faith and the reasonable expectations of insured parties) when coming to a fair and just interpretation of exclusion clauses.

It is suggested, finally, that it may be prudent to re-examine the issues raised by 'post-contractual cherry-picking' in light of the findings of a 1981 report by the Japanese Social Policy Council that examined unfair contractual terms in consumer contracts in Japan (Hasegawa 2005: 100).[7] The report recommended that exclusion clauses should not be applied in cases where the insured party was genuinely unaware that he or she was ill at the time of entering the contract. This approach is entirely consistent with the aims of Articles 644 and 678 of the Japanese Commercial Code, which confine the insurer's right to rescind contracts to situations where the insured party has made false disclosures, or has not disclosed important facts, due to acting either in bad faith or through gross negligence. A subsequent statement by the Japanese Insurance Association (JIA) demonstrated a commitment to bring industry practice into line with the Council's recommendations (Hasegawa 2005: 100).[8] This important undertaking by the JIA, which has never been formally revoked, was overlooked by the Osaka High Court.

ii: Determining the timing of the onset of a 'pre-existing medical condition'
The second point to be established by the 2004 ruling is that, for the purposes of interpreting standard exclusion clauses in Japanese insur-

ance contracts, a genetic predisposition to a disease does not in itself equate to a 'pre-existing medical condition'. Rather, as a matter of legal construction, a person is only deemed to have a pre-existing medical condition when he or she begins to manifest symptoms of the disease or condition outwardly. This symptomatic-asymptomatic distinction means that even under the Osaka High Court's strict approach to the retrospective application of exclusion clauses, an insured party born with a deleterious genetic mutation may be able to claim successfully in relation to the disability caused by the associated disease, if it manifests *after* the commencement of the period of the insurer's contractual liability.

This approach, however, throws the logic of the Court's earlier assertion in point (i) (above) into question. If, as the Court suggested, it is truly necessary to protect the accuracy of actuarial tables by excluding insurance coverage for all high-risk individuals who were exhibiting symptoms of an illness *before* entering into the contract (whether they were aware of their condition or not), then it would also be necessary to extend this policy to exclude high-risk individuals who manifest symptoms *after* the commencement of the contract, as such individuals are equally disruptive to insurers' 'predicted accident occurrence rates'. This inconsistency within the Osaka High Court's reasoning further reinforces the argument that exclusion clauses should only be applied retrospectively, in situations where the insured party has made false disclosures or has not disclosed important facts due to acting either in bad faith or through gross negligence.

iii: Constitutional rights and public morality

The third and perhaps more broadly applicable point to be clarified by the case is that individual rights guaranteed by Article 13 of the Japanese Constitution are not violated by the use of genetic test results in insurance underwriting. Article 13 provides that:

> All of the people shall be respected as individuals. Their right to life, liberty and the pursuit of happiness shall, to the extent that it does not interfere with the public welfare, be the supreme consideration in legislation and other governmental affairs.

X had argued that the use of genetic test results by insurers was an abuse of personal information that would likely discourage people from undergoing tests as part of their healthcare strategy and would therefore impinge upon the terms of Article 13. The Osaka High Court rejected this argument, stating that although some individuals may find themselves disadvantaged due to adverse test results, it may also be the case that other applicants are placed in a more advantageous position with

insurers if results indicate that they are free from genetic predisposi-
tions to disease. When viewed in this light, it was held that the use of
test results as the basis for risk selection by insurance companies did
not infringe upon Constitutional rights, nor was it in violation of more
general concepts of public morality (Yamashita 2004). The court also
added the following statement:

> This case did not concern questions surrounding the provision
> of genetic information for the purposes of entering into an insur-
> ance contract, but as it did concern the use of genetic informa-
> tion to prove the causal relationship with the disease [that mani-
> fested] before the period of liability, it can be thought of as shar-
> ing its roots with the recent debate on how genetic information
> should be handled. Nevertheless, this case related to the problem
> of whether a right to claim insurance money exists when a test
> result is already known, and did not concern the disclosure or
> provision of genetic information. At the current time there are
> not yet any legal regulations regarding the control of genetic in-
> formation. There is therefore no reason to strike out facts that
> are clarified by genetic information under the law of evidence.

Thus, whilst perhaps keeping the door open for the future development
of judicial policy, the 2004 ruling signifies that Japanese insurance
companies are currently free to carry out pre-contractual risk selection
using genetic test results, and can raise premiums or reject applicants
on the basis of their genetic risk status.

The following section argues that the current unchecked, laissez-faire
approach in Japan may be problematic. Stakeholders (including the Japanese government, the insurance industry, medical associations, patient groups and the general public) need to engage with the various issues and work towards the construction of an appropriate regulatory
framework.

Part IV: Genes, free markets and fairness

A: 'Discrimination' and 'actuarial fairness'

One of the key questions that stakeholders need to consider is whether
it is legitimate for insurers to treat applicants less favourably because of
their genetic characteristics. Is this an acceptable form of risk selection,
or alternatively, is it a new and invidious form of 'discrimination'? In
order to respond to this question, we must be clear about how we draw
the boundary between acceptable 'differential treatment' and unjust
'discrimination' (Halldenius 2005; Lemmens 2003).

Discrimination can be defined as: 'differential treatment' (or 'treating less favourably') for 'arbitrary', 'irrational' or 'irrelevant' reasons (Hall-denius 2005; Laurie 2000). When applying this view of discrimination, scrutiny is placed on the relevance of the specific characteristic(s) in question to the given context. Thus, working within this conceptual framework, if we accept that an applicant's medical risk status is relevant in the context of life or health insurance, then we must also accept that, in certain circumstances, treating applicants less favourably on the basis of their genetic test results would not constitute 'discrimination', but would instead be a form of justified 'differential treatment' (Laurie 2000).

This preliminary conclusion would be dependent upon an insurance company being able to demonstrate that the way it had used a specific genetic test result was rational and non-arbitrary, i.e. that it was a proportionate adjustment based on a scientifically sound understanding of the increase in risk indicated by the result. This implements the approach known as 'actuarial fairness' (Ashcroft 2007; Mittra 2007), a requirement lacking in the current Japanese framework. The regulatory system in Australia provides a good example of how actuarial fairness might be achieved in practice.

The Australian Investment and Financial Services Association (IFSA), which represents the Australian insurance industry, has outlined its policy on genetic testing and life insurance (IFSA 2005). The policy clarifies the following points: (1) insurers will not require insurance applicants to undergo genetic testing; (2) insurers will require that applicants make available the results of any previously undertaken genetic tests upon request; (3) insurers will take account of the benefits of special medical monitoring, early medical treatment, compliance with treatment and the likelihood of successful medical treatment when assessing overall risk; and (4) insurers will provide applicants or their medical practitioner with reasons for any adjustment to premiums or policy conditions after assessing an application.

These kinds of minimum basic safeguards should be implemented in Japan. Actuarial fairness would help those who might otherwise be rejected by insurers due to misunderstanding or overestimation of the statistical significance of a particular genetic test (Ashcroft 2007). Furthermore, this approach is logically consistent with the established principle of 'equity', as it simply reflects the idea that the actuarially fair price an individual must pay for premiums is determined by the risk that he or she brings to the insurance pool (Mittra 2007).

Regulators could draw inspiration from the Australian model to construct an actuarially fair governance structure in Japan. Would this approach, however, resolve all the complexities and tensions in this area?

B: The limitations of actuarial fairness

Some commentators have argued that the 'actuarial fairness' approach is something of a narrow paradigm that may clash with broader notions of 'social fairness' in certain instances (Ashcroft 2007). One particular concern is that people's fears about the implications of an adverse test result for their insurance ratings might discourage them from taking tests. Empirical evidence from the UK suggests that one-third of women would not undergo genetic tests for breast cancer if insurers were allowed access to the test result (Mayor 2005). Not only would this disincentive to take tests offend principles of autonomy and self-determination, but in the context of the underutilisation of predictive tests for various forms of cancer, might result in deaths that could otherwise be prevented through close monitoring and early medical interventions (Armstrong et al 2003).

The standard counterargument here is to point out that genetic tests are not unique in this respect; the same basic dynamic is at play when individuals weigh up the pros and cons of undergoing other kinds of predictive medical tests that may impact upon insurance risk status, such as tests for high blood pressure, cholesterol or HIV (Holm 2007). Broadly speaking, this is true, but it is submitted that rather than providing a sound reason for allowing insurers to make use of genetic tests in the same way they currently make use of HIV (and other) tests, this observation merely serves to highlight the broader tension that exists between risk selection principles and the promotion of healthcare interests – a tension which arguably should be resolved in favour of the latter when viable.

A second policy concern surrounding the use of genetic information by Japanese insurers relates to the possibility that it may serve to further solidify and reify the social discrimination towards those suffering from genetic disease that still exists in Japan (Ryder 2005). This is a consideration that may be unwise to ignore completely.

It is therefore suggested that there are good reasons why Japanese stakeholders should at least consider looking beyond the actuarial fairness model to assess the viability of other frameworks that could help further the public interest in this area without causing undue disruption to the Japanese insurance industry.

Part V: Beyond actuarial fairness: suggestions for balancing public and private interests

One approach that could be adopted as a means to reconcile commercial concerns with healthcare policy and other objectives in Japan is the 'ceiling approach' used in the United Kingdom. The UK model has evolved through dialogue between government and the Association of British Insurers (ABI), a body which represents the British insurance industry. Following discussions and negotiation with the Genetics and Insurance Committee (GAIC), the ABI published a Concordat and Moratorium on Genetics and Insurance in 2005, which seeks to strike a pragmatic balance between public and private interests (Department of Health & ABI 2005). A primary feature of the UK approach is that insurance companies have agreed not to use any genetic test results unless the significance and accuracy of those specific tests has first been assessed and approved by the GAIC. So far, only one test, for Huntington's disease, has received GAIC approval.

The Concordat, which has been extended until 2014, ensures that insurance applicants will not be asked to disclose the results of predictive genetic tests for life insurance policies with a value of under £ 500,000, or for critical illness policies of a value of less than £ 300,000. It is stated that over 97 per cent of all life and health insurance policies in the UK are for far less than these amounts. If, however, applicants wish to purchase insurance policies worth more than these threshold values, they will be asked to disclose the results of genetic tests, and insurers will be free to act upon adverse test results by raising premiums or denying coverage. Individuals will not be required to undergo genetic tests as part of their applications. Furthermore, results arising from genetic research projects need not be disclosed to insurers. Finally, where an individual's family medical history suggests a high risk of genetic disease, a test result indicating that an applicant does not carry a genetic susceptibility can be used to allow that applicant to contract on standard terms.

The ABI seems fairly unconcerned about the limited financial losses that it may suffer under the Concordat, and this is likely to be because there are so few people in the UK with a predisposition for Huntington's disease (Thomas 2007). The overall commercial impact of a ceiling approach in Japan would likely be smaller still, as the insurance market is larger and the prevalence rates of Huntington's disease and most other serious genetic diseases are generally lower than those found in Western countries (Mutō 2000).

It is important to note that the UK Concordat does not guarantee access to private insurance. The narrow definition of genetic tests used in the Concordat, which only applies to predictive genetic tests that examine the structure of chromosomes (cytogenetic tests) or detect abnormal patterns in the DNA of specific genes (molecular tests), means that insurers can still make use of non-genetic medical test results, such as blood or urine tests for cholesterol, prostate cancer, liver function or diabetes, or indeed family history. This information can be used to assess risk, raise premiums, change policy terms or decline coverage to certain individuals. As previously mentioned, family medical history is not normally requested by insurers in Japan (Miyachi 2005: 112), and this might mean that if a ceiling approach were implemented in Japan, application outcomes for individuals with a family history of illness might be somewhat more favourable than for similarly situated individuals in the UK.

An alternative approach could be to develop 'guaranteed issue' private insurance products that may be purchased without the need for medical examinations or even the disclosure of any health-related information. Though at first glance this might seem to be a utopian aspiration that ignores fundamental principles of private insurance, 'guaranteed issue' health insurance products are already commercially available in Japan, and have been designed for and sold to the middle-aged and the elderly, who may be excluded from purchasing standard insurance products due to health complications (Otomo 2005).

A number of restrictions and limitations are put in place on guaranteed issue policies to reduce the risks undertaken by the insurer. Mechanisms include significantly higher insurance premiums, reduced levels of payouts and the exclusion of liability for any illness manifesting prior to the commencement of the policy. Guaranteed issue products therefore allow even high-risk applicants to receive basic private health insurance coverage, though at a much higher price than that paid by applicants in good health. To the extent that guaranteed issue insurance products are available (and affordable) to the majority of the Japanese population, people will be unlikely to be deterred from undergoing valuable genetic tests. The Japanese insurance industry could also consider developing guaranteed issue products for life insurance and long-term nursing care, perhaps with the benefit of subsidies from the Japanese government if necessary.

Conclusion

The Japanese government and the Japanese insurance industry have been notably slow to address the issues raised by genetic testing in the context of insurance. The fact that the first legal dispute concerning the use of genetic test results by insurers has already reached the Japanese courts suggests that it is now time for stakeholders to commit to constructing a proper regulatory framework. This paper has argued that at least minimum safeguards of actuarial fairness should be established in Japan, and has also suggested that there are valid reasons why regulators should further consider the viability of other models that would help balance commercial interests with public concerns.

On a final note, it is perhaps appropriate to place the current debate about genetic tests and access to private insurance in Japan in its proper perspective. The problems raised by genetic tests are not entirely new. Rather, genetic testing simply highlights and exacerbates two pre-existing tensions in the operation of insurance markets. First, the current discussion shows that the 'privatisation of welfare' is in itself inherently problematic, as a certain degree of exclusion is always likely to occur in commercial markets (Mittra 2007). Second, the problem of individuals electing not to undergo genetic tests or other predictive tests (such as HIV tests) because of the fear that it will render them uninsurable illustrates the conflict that can arise between the principles of risk selection and healthcare interests. It is hoped that these difficult, broader issues may also be addressed in Japan and other countries over the coming years.

Acknowledgements

I would like to express my sincere thanks to Associate Professor Itsuko Yamaguchi and Associate Professor Noritaka Yamashita for their kind assistance in locating Japanese research materials, and also to Dr Margaret Sleeboom-Faulkner and Professor Graeme Laurie for their helpful comments and suggestions on earlier drafts of this paper. Any mistakes are the sole responsibility of the author.

Notes

1   Section 101(6)(A) of GINA defines genetic information as meaning, with respect to any individual, information about: (i) such individual's genetic tests, (ii) the genetic tests of family members of such individual, and (iii) the manifestation of a disease or disorder in family members of such individual.
2   As of 25 June 2008, 100 yen = US $ 0.93.
3   Kobe District Court, 2000, (Wa) No. 575. Judgement issued on 18 June 2003.
4   Osaka High Court, 2003 (Ne) No.2260. Judgement issued on 27 May 2004.
5   Supreme Court of Japan, 27 October 1989, *Bunken Seimei Hoken Hanreishū* 6, 103.
6   See *Zeller v. British Caymanian Insurance Co Ltd* [2008] All ER (D) 219 (Jan); *Cook v. Financial Insurance* [1998] 1 W.L.R. 1765; *Econimedes v. Commercial Assurance Co* [1998] QB 587; *Joel v. Law Union and Crown Insurance Co.* [1908] 2 K.B. 863.
7   See the 1981 *Citizens Life Advisory Board* 'Fair Revision of Consumer Contract Terms'.
8   *Seimei Hoken Kyoukai Hō*, Vol. 62, No.2, Art.67

9 Genetic Testing for Duchenne Muscular Dystrophy in China: Vulnerabilities among Chinese Families

Suli Sui and Margaret Sleeboom-Faulkner

Introduction

In China, about 650,000 affected boys suffer from Duchenne muscular dystrophy[1] (Chinese Red Cross Foundation 2005). Duchenne muscular dystrophy (DMD), the most common childhood muscular dystrophy, is a lethal X-linked genetic disorder, which affects approximately 1 in 4500 live male births (Garner-Medwin & Sharples 1989). DMD carriers pass it on to one-half of their sons – which means 50 per cent of male offspring will be affected – and one-half of their daughters, who become carriers (Harper 2004: 100). This chapter concerns the consequences of the application of genetic testing and genetic counselling on this sex-linked genetic disorder. Genetic counselling and testing on DMD has important implications for reproductive decisions and life planning decisions, which are also affected in China by economic conditions, access to the healthcare system, the Chinese family-planning policy, Chinese reproductive views and Chinese culture. This case study of DMD aims to acquire a better understanding of economic difficulties, psychological distress, self-contempt and family stigma that families are confronted with in Chinese contexts. Based on the complexity of conditions of families with DMD, this study rethinks some related social issues such as genetic discrimination, the distribution of health resources, the reliability of medical information, the access to basic knowledge and of medical treatment for prevailing genetic disorders, the impact of genetic technology on reproductive decision-making, social support and help for vulnerable groups.

This chapter is the result of an empirical survey conducted from September 2007 to February 2008 in China. During the survey, the first author collected basic information about genetic testing on DMD in China through archival study and Internet research. The original data are obtained from interviews and participant observation. During fieldwork, the first author interviewed five geneticists and six doctors working in a clinic as genetic counsellors, and sat in at two sessions of genetic counselling in both the paediatric department and maternity department of Beijing Xiehe Hospital. The sessions target genetic disorders in general, not just DMD, but one session usually includes two or three consultants of families with DMD from all over the country. As a 'novice doctor' (jianxi yisheng),[2] the first author collected first-hand information on the practice of genetic counselling on DMD. Such experience provided access to boys with DMD and their families. The method of deep interview was used for ten families with DMD, and four families with DMD were selected as case studies, with which regular contact was maintained. The research method of participant observation yielded a better understanding of the daily routine and the problems that families with DMD experience in daily life.

The practice of genetic counselling and testing for Duchenne muscular dystrophy in China

Although there is no cure or effective treatment available for DMD, an early diagnosis is ideally made, primarily to offer genetic counselling, and, where possible, prenatal diagnosis. When diagnosis of DMD takes place, the family is warned that DMD is an inherited disorder and that the sisters and cousins of the affected boy have a high risk of being carriers. Improving the identification of carriers is aimed at reducing the number of boys with DMD being born in affected families, as is the case in Europe (Emery 1991). In China, it is the genetic counselling clinic, usually located in the paediatric department or/and maternity department of a hospital, that offers genetic testing for diagnosis. For the prenatal genetic counselling and testing, it is usually in the genetic clinic of the maternity department, because the test sample and the amniotic fluid are collected by amniocentesis, an operation usually performed by a maternity doctor in the prenatal clinic. Guidelines for Genetic Counselling promulgated by the Chinese Ministry of Health (MOH) in 2003 regulate the basic requests, principles and procedures of genetic counselling in China. According to these guidelines, genetic counselling should be offered by clinicians who have a knowledgeable background of genetics. In practice, the counsellors in the genetic counselling clinic usually are clinicians, such as paediatricians and obstetricians, with a background in genetics. In China, genetic counselling is combined with testing, and it is the doctor who works as a counsellor, prescribing the testing for clients/patients. Because of the advanced nature of the technology of genetic testing on DMD, the qualification should be authorized by the Provincial Health Department.[3] There are only a few hospitals that are well known for their genetics departments.

Among them, Beijing Xiehe Hospital, Hunan Xiangya Hospital and Shenyang Medical University No.2 Hospital are authorised to offer DMD genetic testing. Most of the families coming to the counselling clinic obtain information on access to genetic counselling/diagnosis from doctors in their local hospital.

In the genetic counselling clinic, collecting genetic information is the first important step. In counselling practice in the UK, general strategy demands that at least basic details for both sides of the family are taken, even in a dominantly inherited disorder clearly originating from one side. Taking histories from both sides may help to avoid feelings of guilt or blame resting exclusively on one member of a couple. This may always be an important factor, but it is particularly important in some cultures and social situations (Harper 2004: 7-8). This view is also accepted by Chinese genetic counsellors and is applied in particular for X-linked inherited disorders such as DMD. In the counselling clinic for DMD, doctors make efforts to avoid spreading feelings of guilt and blame among husband and wife. Usually during the first consultation of the counselling clinic, symptoms of the boy suspected of having DMD are checked, the disease history of both partners' families is taken, and the doctor provides an initial diagnosis. This initial step is complemented with genetic testing for confirmation. During the consultation, the doctor will explain some basic knowledge of DMD in simple terms, though the doctor usually does not mention the X-linked inherited character to the couples directly. Usually, in practice, the doctor emphasises that spontaneous mutations also can result in the birth of boys affected with DMD, avoiding the issues of 'responsibility' for the boy's affliction. During counselling sessions on DMD, the doctor working as a genetic counsellor in the clinic also takes into account the position of women and the stability of the couple's marriage and their family. The survey among geneticists also showed that genetic counselling on X-link disorders should try to play down (danhua, a literal translation to English is 'de-salinate') the issue of 'individual responsibility' for the genetic disorder.

Doctor Shi, a geneticist cum doctor working in the genetic counselling clinic, exemplifies genetic counsellors in China:

> In counselling a family with DMD, I usually do not choose to directly tell the couple, especially the husband, about the inherited character of DMD. There have already been some examples where, after the husband realises that the boy's disease is a result of his wife's genes, he blames the wife and divorces her. Usually the wife feels guilty and blames herself for the condition. If the husband requires divorce, she has no choice. You know, it is very miserable for a single mother with an affected child. Considering

this, I sometimes think that it is preferable to use a 'fog bomb' (*yanwu dan*, literally 'smoke bomb', a concept used to describe 'making hazy' or 'to cover up'), especially in the case of families that come from rural areas, where the Chinese traditional 'boy-preference' prevails compaed with urban regions. If the family does not ask, I don't tell them. But if they do ask, I give them a 'fog bomb', as if either of them could have been the 'cause', or as if there could have been a mutation. In fact, there is a possibility of genetic mutation, and it is difficult to give a definite answer. I hope that the couple become mental prepared, and understand that the most important thing is to face the facts instead of feeling guilt or blaming the other. (Interview, 17 October 2007. Transl. SS)

In practice, the first consultation in the genetic counselling clinic usually ends with the prescription of genetic testing, and the blood sample will be collected from the affected boy and both parents. The doctor suggests that the couple come to the genetic counselling clinic for a second consultation, usually two months later, and at that time the genetic testing result is ready. For the second consultation, if the result diagnosis is DMD, the doctor will give directions on how to take care of a boy with DMD. Stretching, massage and low-impact sports are usually recommended by doctor to the parent of such a boy. According to the family pedigree, the doctor gives advice that the female members of the family, who have a high risk of being carriers, ought to take the test. The doctor also advises the couple to make sure prenatal genetic testing is available before they plan another pregnancy and take a prenatal genetic test during the next pregnancy.

Cases selected for understanding complexity conditions of families with Duchenne muscular dystrophy

This study is based upon conversations with approximately thirty DMD consultancy clients, including affected boys, carrier women and their families. From these, three cases were chosen as case studies and one, based on Internet research, was added. The four cases were selected to offer insight into the variety of the circumstances in which families of boys with DMD have to make decisions, the complexity of conditions in which such families live their daily lives, and the vulnerability of these families in China. The four case studies are analysed in the following sections.

Case 1: Mrs Sun wants a genetic test
This case concerns the decision-making regarding the termination of pregnancy and the expectations of this family about the genetic technology. The case shows that family history did not get the attention it deserved in this family.

Mrs Sun, a seven-month pregnant woman from Qingyang, a small city in Gansu province, applied for prenatal genetic testing on DMD. Her application was rejected because it was too late to take amniocentesis at seven months' gestation, which is very dangerous for both mother and foetus. In practice, amniocentesis is commonly used as a measure to collect samples for prenatal genetic testing. Amniocentesis is performed at 10 to 20 weeks' gestation in current clinical application in China. Mrs Sun and her husband made the decision to take a carrier test and decided to terminate the pregnancy if the test indicated her to be a carrier of DMD. Although one of her older brothers, two cousins and one nephew died as a result of DMD, she was not aware of her family history regarding DMD. She ascribes her little knowledge about DMD in her family history to the large size of her family and to having almost no memory of her deceased elder brother. When the son of one of her cousins, a four-year-old boy, started to show the symptoms of DMD and was diagnosed after taking a genetic test, she panicked and went to the genetic counselling clinic to ask for a test. The boy, from Quzi town, Huan County in Gansu province, is the only affected living male in this big family. His father and mother work as 'migrant farm workers' in Guangzhou. 'Migrant farm workers' (*nongmin gong*) are farmers who have temporary jobs in the city. His parents left him with his grandparent. Now, Mr Sun, an older brother of Mrs Sun, who is a surgeon in a hospital in Beijing, hopes that the genetic testing can help to eliminate this disorder from his big family by preventing the birth of affected boys and new carriers. (Interview with Ms Sun, her husband and her brother on 16 and 20 November 2007)

Case 2: Mrs Lu and her husband want to have a daughter
This case illustrates 'gender preference' in reproduction, the social isolation of boys with DMD, the psychological pressure and the difficulties the families of such boys face in China.

Mrs Lu is from Gaozuo Town, Suining County, in Jiangsu Province. Mrs Lu is the mother of a 9-year-old DMD-afflicted boy. Two years ago, this family took a genetic test in Xiehe Hospital, and the boy was diagnosed with DMD. Now the boy can no longer walk well. His situation gets worse when he wears thick winter clothes in cold weather. Every day, his father or mother carries him to school and gets him home using a manual tricycle (*renli sanlun che*). On this occasion, Mrs Lu came to the genetic counselling clinic when she was twelve weeks pregnant. She and her husband fervently hoped for a girl and decided to take a prenatal genetic test in Xiehe hospital. One month after the test sample was collected through amniocentesis,[4] they received the test result that showed the foetus to be female. The couple was very happy when they heard the result and they do not greatly care whether their future daughter is a carrier or not. Mrs Lu and her husband know about the inherited nature of DMD. Mrs Lu has told her sisters and cousins about the inheritability of DMD and the possibility of their being a carrier, but they do not believe her and do not take it seriously. (Interviews with Mrs Lu and her husband on 27 November 2007 in Xiehe Hospital, on 6 December 2007 when Mrs Lu had amniocentesis in Xiehe Hospital and on 16 December 2007 in their home)

Case 3: Liang and his family feel stigmatised
This case shows how DMD is intimately linked with the family-planning policy and the daily lives of families that carry DMD.

A DMD-affected boy named Liang, an 8-year-old primary school student, lives in Hongni village, Wulian County, Shandong Province. His mother, Mrs Yang, is 45 years of age. Liang, who was diagnosed with DMD after taking a genetic test, clearly has problems moving and standing steadily. Liang has an old sister named Xiu who is 23 and temporarily works in Rizhao city. The doctor advised her to undertake a carrier test. She has already reached the legal age, which is 20, for women to get married in China. Liang's father, grandfather and grandmother all did not know clearly about the hereditary character of DMD. Mrs Yang had another son who was younger than the daughter. After she gave birth to this boy, she had to undergo sterilisation by joining the oviducts (jieza), in agreement with the family-planning policy. Unfortunately, this boy drowned when he was three years old. It was a severe shock for the family. After undergoing an operation to 'unjoin the oviduct' (shu luan guan fu tong), the mother conceived again and gave birth to Liang. Now the mother is too old to have another pregnancy. The economic situation of this family, with a DMD affected boy in a small village, is difficult. Apart from their financial hardships, the mother suffers severely due to self-condemnation and feelings of guilt. Moreover, the family also experiences discrimination in the village and feels stigmatised as family with a disabled boy. (Interviews with the mother and sister on 9 December 2007 and subsequently)

Case 4: Ms Xue and her sons persevere
This case study draws on information from the Internet and a film, which is based on the true story of a family from Xian, the capital city of Shanxi province. Ms Xue, a single mother, has DMD-affected twins

named Gold Bean and Silver Bean (*Jindou* and *Yingdou*: 'Bean' is used as name in Chinese denoting 'baby' or 'sonny'). Now the boys are adolescents. Ms Xue divorced when she was 31 and the boys were six. After her divorce, she brought up and looked after the two affected boys. In order to dedicate herself to the boys entirely and to avoid anguish for the boys, she decided not to remarry. Ms Xue strictly ensures the boys take exercise every day, such as a five-kilometre walk. She gives massage to the boys and helps them to do sit-ups every day by pushing their backs, because they cannot do this themselves. She tried to seek alternative treatment for DMD, which actually had little effect. The boys easily catch flu due to their low resistance, so that she spends much energy and time caring for them. Ms Xue, who works in a textile mill, therefore cannot afford to work full time. The family lives on her small income and often faces financial difficulties. The experience of the family attracted public attention, after which their story was written down as a play and was filmed as a television drama named *Loving You Using My Life* (*Yong wo de shengming qu ai ni*).

These four cross-sectional cases offer insight into the circumstances and experiences of families with DMD in China. The next sections will address and analyse social issues linked to DMD and DMD genetic knowledge.

The social and political framework of choice of DMD families in China

Based on the case studies, this section will analyse the vulnerability of DMD families and related issues such as the social stigma of the DMD-affected boys and their families, the lack of welfare support and social help for the families of boys with DMD, and the impact of living with DMD-affected boys on reproductive decision-making and reproductive views.

Lack of effective treatment

Twenty years after the discovery of the DMD gene in 1988, an effective medical treatment is still not available (Urtizberea et al 2003). Although DMD is present from conception, boys with this disorder appear normal at birth. It is when they begin to walk that discrepancies are often noted. In most cases, the child walks with a 'waddling gait', tends to tip-toe, and has overdeveloped calves. Later, climbing stairs becomes challenging (Cwik & Brooke 1996). When the symptoms appear, parents initially do not think it is a serious problem and think that the child is just a late developer. Ms Lu in Case 2 said when she found her son walked slowly, she thought it was common that a boy learns to walk later than a girl, or maybe that her son did not take enough calcium and vitamins. She became worried about the 'walking problem' after she found her son could not climb the stairs like the other boys of the same age. In fact, most families with an affected boy share a similar experience. They come to hospital in the hopes of getting treatment. When parents find out that this is a lethal disorder and that no effective treatment is available, they usually react with feelings of disbelief, denial, anger, anguish and anxiety (DMD Forum 2001). Ms Xue, the mother of the twins in Case 4, remembers the way she felt:

> I felt like the sky was falling down on me (*tian ta le*), I nearly lost my consciousness at that moment, like a huge thunder hit my head. The diagnosis result was like a death penalty sentence. I cannot believe my sons will die. ... Why am I so unlucky? Why are my sons so unlucky? Why? (transl. SS)

Ms Yang, in Case 3, had a similar reaction: 'I felt so cold. Just like I dropped into an ice cave (*bing kulong*). My mind became blank (*yipian kongbai*). If this disease can be cured, I will try to collect money to treat him, even sell the last thing in my home (*zaguo maitie*).

Many families try to find an alternative treatment, although the doctors have told them clearly that no medical treatment can cure DMD at this time. They believe what the doctor said but they fervently hope that maybe something else would work. In the clinic, some parents begged the doctor to allow their son to become a human subject in clinical experiments as soon as new therapy for DMD might be developed. Some families turned to traditional Chinese medicine. In fact, according to a pilot study carried out in Beijing on ten DMD-affected boys treated with traditional Chinese medicine at various stages of their disease course, it is not possible to draw any definitive conclusions regarding the beneficial effect of Chinese traditional herbal medicine in patients with DMD. It seems as if the benefit, if any, is minimal (Urtizberea et al 2003). Also, parents of DMD-affected boys who are tempted to get access to these drugs often are not informed of their effects and potential hazards, although the potential toxicity of some of these Chinese traditional medicines has clearly been demonstrated elsewhere in other conditions (Chan & Critchley 1996; Critchley et al 2000). In fact, there are some, usually little known, hospitals that boast in exaggerated advertisements special treatments for incurable diseases such as DMD (Chen 2005). The advertisements attract people, including those from remote rural areas, whose family members suffer from incurable diseases, such as cancer and DMD. The strong desire for treatment easily misleads DMD-affected families into spending money, worsening their financial situation. One interviewee in such a situation expressed her feeling of helplessness:

If I do not try, I will feel guilty towards my son. The advertisement said that the treatment is effective. Maybe there is a possibility. Maybe it will be helpful. I am not rich, but I will try at least once. Anyway, I think that the treatment will not make things worse. I only want to make every possible effort (*si ma dang huo ma yi*, a literal translation to English is 'to treat a dead horse like an alive one'). (transl. SS)

Psychological distress and heavy burden for the parents and family

Parents of boys with DMD say they experience depression and emotional anguish. Because some parents view their child as an extension of themselves, they are apt to feel that such a disorder reflects upon them. They feel grief, and a feeling of guilt is a common response to grief. Particularly, mothers with a defective X chromosome have the added burden of knowing that they are most likely the unwitting carriers of the gene responsible for the disorder (Rubin 1987). As the disease progresses, mothers may develop an attitude of self-blame and struggle with guilt regarding the child's condition. Also, the long-term and escalating nature of DMD creates an increasing burden on families as the disease progresses. Caring for a family member with a severe chronic illness has been associated with increased family stress, diminished health for caretakers and an increased financial burden (Wang & Barnard 2004). Family members must provide increasing assistance with activities of daily life, eventually having to carry them out completely for the affected child. Long-term care needs may increase the financial burden on the family, particularly if one of parents needs to forego employment to care for the child (Chen & Clark 2007). As a single mother with two sons who need her care, Ms Xue in Case 4 has a heavy financial burden and psychological stress:

When I am short of money – I only had 20 Yuan (about 2 Euro) – I do not know what to do. At that time, I even planned to sell my kidney, although I know it is illegal to sell human organs. Often, I want to cry, shout, or sing loudly. I even considered committing suicide together with my sons, so as to finish it all (*yi liao bai liao*). Sometimes I cannot sleep at night and stand in the dark, smoking cigarette after cigarette. In that year, when my sons were 12 years old, I started to lose my hair. I shed a lot every day. In addition, every day I accompanied my sons for five-kilometre walks and I engaged in massage and stretching exercises for my sons. I often feel my body and soul are all exhausted (*xinli jiaocui*). (Transl. SS)

Ms Yang, in Case 3, also feels she is under the pressure of guilt, depression and anxiety:

> I feel life is bleak and colourless. Watching my son walking in that way, thinking he will be unable to walk and that he will die, my heart hurts so much, like it is being pricked by a sharp needle (*xin ru zhen za*). If I could, I would like to bare the pain of my son [she said crying]. It is my fault, and I feel so bad and feel so sorry (*dui bu zhu*) for my son and my husband. If my husband wants to divorce me, I have nothing to say. My son is still young and he does not understand his disease, and I do not want him to know more. I only hope he can be happy. (Transl. SS)

From Ms Xue's and Ms Yang's narratives, we can understand the heavy psychological burden of the mothers.

Stigma and discrimination against families with Duchenne muscular dystrophy

Ervin Goffman, a well-known sociologist, defined the concept of stigma as denoting an attribute that is deeply discrediting, which reduces the possessor in our minds from a whole and usual person to a tainted, discounted one (Latz 1981). The attribute that stigmatises one type of possessor can confirm the usualness of another, and therefore is neither creditable nor discreditable as a thing in itself (Goffman 1986: 3). The 'abomination of the body' is a type of stigma, consisting of various physical deformities, disabilities and chronic diseases. People use specific stigma terms, such as cripple and moron, in daily discourse as a source of metaphor and imagery (Goffman 1986: 5). In practice, persons suffering from a severe illness and their close family members are often socially stigmatised (Sartorius 1997). A popular view in China considers severe illness, to a certain extent, to be punishment for an ancestor's misbehaviour or for the family's current misconduct, which is called 'religious punishment' (*zongjiao chengfa*) or 'pre-existence retribution' (*qianshi baoying*) (Lin & Lin 1980; Wang & Zhang 2002; Liu 2006). This view, which is a popular explanation of pathogenesis based on religion and superstition, sometimes is used to stigmatise families with severe handicaps, causing conflict and dissatisfaction. Such stigma and discrimination make the disabled feel distressed. In fact, it is very difficult for the disabled to lead a 'normal' life, so that it is challenging for the disabled to get married, and the disability sets them apart from their friends and neighbours (Kohrman 1999). As a lethal inherited disorder, DMD instils fear in people. The long process of progressive weakening of the patient, and the late-onset genetic nature of the disease, resulting in early death, intensifies the stigmatisation of the family. Stigma and discrimination teach family members self-contempt and guilt, isolating them from the community. The DMD-affected family members interviewed all felt that their family was suffering from the stigma and discrimination. Mr Sun, the elder brother of Ms Sun in Case 1, said his childhood was full of painful memories of having an affected young brother:

> Sometimes several boys in the neighbourhood followed him, simulating his walking style, mocking him, and calling him 'cripple' (que zi). This illness is monstrous and strange. One of my uncles died from it. My family was the target of gossip in the community, which enjoyed chatting about my family. Some words, like 'misconduct', 'sin', 'retribution' and so on (zuo nie, zui guo, bao ying, shenmode) would eventually reach the ears of my family. My family could not do anything to stop it and did not dare to do anything because we were afraid that the gossip would worsen.

> I am so lucky to be the one who is unaffected. Now, I have drawn a pedigree and found those who are at risk of being a carrier and developing the disease. I will try to contact them and offer them money to take a test. I hope no newly affected boys and no new carriers will be born to my family. Let this damned illness disappear from my family. (Transl. SS)

Ms Lu, in Case 2, and her husband are also afraid of stigma and discrimination:

> The symptoms of my son are getting obvious and we cannot keep it secret, but we do not say more about this illness to others except to our very close relative. We are afraid of gossip. We are very cautious and scrupulous to avoid offending anyone. In school, several classmates laughed at my son and he feels bad. The only thing we can do is to implore the teacher to pay more attention. (Transl. SS)

Ms Yang also feels that she and her family are severely stigmatised:

> We cannot hold our heads high in the village. We lost one son, and we will lose this one, too. A family without a son is despised in this village. Some people think our family is cursed by a devil. In our village, usually, a matchmaker will come to a girl's home to propose a candidate for marriage (ti qin) when she approaches

the age of 20. My daughter is 23, and no matchmaker came for her. (Transl. SS)

The girl, daughter of Ms Yang, expressed her feeling about this:

> I feel pity for (*kelian*) my little brother and my mother. I do not want others to know about the situation of my little brother and my carrier state. I keep it secret in the place where I work. I have no boyfriend at present. If I have a boyfriend, I do not know whether I will tell him my carrier state or not. Maybe I will tell him. I think I should not cheat and it cannot be kept secret forever. Many of my classmates are already married. You know, in our small place early marriage is common. Now I do not think more about this. What will be will be (*shun qi ziran*).

One interviewee in this study, a carrier of DMD, also narrated her experience. She said that the parents of her boyfriend strongly set themselves against the relationship between her and their son when they found out about her carrier status, and finally her boyfriend separated from her. This case showed a severe stigmatisation of the DMD-affected family, worsened by popular superstition.

Implication for reproductive decision-making

Gender preference in Chinese views on reproduction is not unusual, and expresses a strong male bias (Zheng 2004). This preference is expressed in the burning of incense for ancestors, a revived tradition increasingly prevalent in China. In Chinese traditional reproductive views, only the male is treated as family offspring, called 'burning incense' (*xiang huo*, in Chinese it means the son/sons in a family) (Liu 2005), for traditional custom prescribes that only a son can hold a memorial ceremony for the ancestor. So, 'burning incense' used in Chinese especially means the male offspring of a family. However, because boys are symptomatic for DMD, the DMD-affected families have strong preferences for having a girl rather than a boy. Ms Sun's words in Case 1 illustrate this:

> If only this foetus were female, I could unburden my mind and relax. But I already know he is a boy. If I am a carrier, there is a 50 per cent risk that he will be affected. I cannot or dare not take such a high risk. You know I hurt a lot. My baby is already a little person now. I can feel him moving every day. It is so great to feel his action. I am such a cruel mama. I really hope that my baby is a girl; if it were, nobody could persuade me to give her up. (Transl. SS)

And Ms Xue, mother of the twins with DMD:

> My family was very proud of the birth of my twin sons before the boys developed symptoms. When the boys were 1 month old (*man yue*), their grandmother boiled two hundred eggs and co-loured them red after which they offered two to every family in the community. Our neighbours and friends all admired me very much. But now, they all feel sorry for me. Sometimes I speculate about what if my twin sons were twin girls, or even just one girl. ... But life cannot be changed. (Transl. SS)

Ms Lu expressed her joy when she found out that her foetus was a girl: 'When I just conceived this time, I always prayed. I hoped that God would give me a girl. I also had a strong feeling this foetus is a girl. I am really happy to know she is a girl. I do not care if she is a carrier or not.'

It is no doubt that boy-preference is the major factor influencing the Chinese couple's expectation and action for reproduction. In some rural areas, sex-selective abortion is also the main reason for the skewed sex ratio in China, particularly in rural areas (Li 2004). In China, one of the main issues in birth policymaking is that many second children were allowed as exceptions to the one-child ideal. The upshot was that about half of the rural couples whose first child was a daughter were al-lowed to try again for a son. This birth policy in rural areas remains in effect in the early twenty-first century, subject to informal debate, but is evidently not yet ready for formal reconsideration (Greenhalgh 2005). The exceptions in the one-child policy imply and represent the son-pre-ference in China. In the context of DMD, sex selection is reversed.

Social isolation of the affected boys
Children with disabilities are limited in their activities in society. Ac-cording to research on issues of the disabled in China, there are an esti-mated 2.15 million children with a disability who are not receiving schooling. However, 76 per cent would be physically able to attend school, but have no opportunity to do so. Furthermore, only 5 per cent of young people with a disability live in the cities, where they might at-tend special schools for the disabled, which are rare in China. This leaves the majority, who live in the countryside, uncatered for (Stratford & Ng 2000). Similarly, children with DMD in this study have little op-portunity to join their peer group in school, because of walking difficul-ties, which make them more likely to be socially isolated.

This research on DMD-affected families suggests that they also ex-perience great social isolation from the community. For instance, par-ents report that their boy does not like going to school and wants to stay at home to watch TV instead. Ms Yang complained: 'My son spends much more time watching TV. Sometimes he sits before the TV set for a long time, even though the programmes are not interesting. I think he is getting more sensitive as he is getting older. He is afraid to get hurt outside and tries to avoid it.'

The father in Case 2 also reported that his son had become quiet:

> My son does not like to play with other children even when they invite him and are friendly to him. He likes watching TV, and sometimes draws pictures. I think that he feels inferior when he plays with other children. You know, he cannot run or even walk properly. (Transl. SS)

Examples of the social isolation of boys with DMD show that such boys feel unsafe and feel that the community does not accept them.

Support from society
In China, there are several Internet communities for 'muscle illness patients' (ji ji huazhe). These Internet communities, such as 'Going with you' (jingcai tongxing, http://www.jingcai.org) and 'window for muscle atrophy' (ji weisuo zhi chuang, http://www.bbs.chinajws.com) offer virtual space for patients and their family to communicate and share their experiences. Also there are several websites that offer general genetic knowledge and answer questions online, which is called 'counselling on-line' (zaixian zixun), such as 'muscle atrophy web' (ji weisuo wang, http://www.ci123.com) and 'genetic question and answer web' (yichuan wenda wang, http:// www. gcnet.org). The resources provided through the Internet to some extent are helpful to patients with DMD and their families. But in China, most rural areas and small towns have no access to the Internet. For most villagers, the Internet is far away from their lives, as they do not know how to use a computer in the first place.

In China, in December 2005, the Red Cross established the DMD Fund, called 'kindness from an angel' (tianshi zhi en) (Zhang 2005). The purpose of the fund is to help DMD-affected boys. At its launch, the fund was valued at one hundred thousand renminbi (about 10,000 euros). It had been donated by a video company and contributed to the treatment and care of DMD-affected twins Gold Bean and Silver Bean, on whose case the film Using My Life to Love You (yong wo de shengming qu ai ni) was modelled. Afterwards, the fund was only able to help one boy with DMD in Beijing with a donation of ten thousand renminbi (about 1,000 euros) in 2007 (Chinese Red Cross Foundation, 2007). None of the DMD-affected families involved in this study had heard of the fund, and they did not regard applying to it as a viable option.

Conclusion

Based on the cases of the four DMD-affected families and their narration of personal experiences and feelings, this paper focuses on the socio-economic aspects of the DMD-affected family, and analyses related social issues in Chinese contexts, such as reproductive decision-making, family stigma and social discrimination, and the difficulties the families affected by DMD encountered in the Chinese contexts. In China today, DMD-affected families are not only undergoing economic hardships, which are caused by the cost of ineffective treatment and energy and time spent on the attentive assistance for DMD-affected children, but are also facing heavy psychological pressure as a result of family stigma mainly coming from the view of 'pre-existence retribution' as a explanation of pathogenesis based on religion and superstition. Meanwhile, the Chinese cultural values attached to healthy offspring increase the psychological burden, especially for the mothers, who usually are strongly self-condemnatory and are blamed by family members. Families affected by DMD are vulnerable, and the existing social discrimination aggravates their vulnerability. Additionally, social welfare and support, due to the lack of accessibility and effect, does not play a full role in reducing the vulnerability of these families.

Other issues that should be explored are the present non-professional modes of genetic counselling and its implications in Chinese contexts. Therefore, more social-scientific research is needed to understand the application of genetic technology and the social implications in this field.

Notes

1   Duchenne muscular dystrophy is a recessive disease. The female is carrier and transmits the disease genetically to offspring, but does not develop it. DMD is caused by the lack of dystrophin, which is a protein found in the cell membrane of muscles. Boys are normal at birth and only begin to show signs of the muscle wasting disease when they are 3 or 4 years old. They experience increasing difficulty walking because of progressive weakness with loss of ambulation and are often wheelchair bound by 11-12 years old. The muscle deterioration is continuous and they usually die in their late teens, or early twenties, because no effective treatment is yet available (Parsons et al 2000).

2   Noviciate doctors in China usually are medical students who are in the last year of university education. Clinical experience for noviciate doctors is compulsory before graduation. Thanks to the introduction of one respected professor and consent from the doctors and patients, I got chance to carry out my survey as a 'noviciate doctor' in a clinic.

3   According to the *Measures for the administration of prenatal diagnosis technology*, which is a document promulgated by the MOH in 2003, hospitals/healthcare providers certified only by the Provincial Health Department can practice prenatal genetic diagnosis.

4   Amniocentesis is a procedure in which a small sample of amniotic fluid is drawn out of the uterus through a needle inserted into the abdomen. The fluid is then analysed to detect genetic abnormalities in the foetus or to determine the sex of the foetus.

10 Ramification of Choice?

Ethical, Cultural and Social Dimensions of Sex Selection in China

Ole Döring

Ethics and choice in context

Attempts to 'choose' or determine our children's sex raise questions for cultural analysis in the area of bioethics. Beyond revealing value orientations and the situation of discourse, such choices can indicate socio-economic conditions. symptomatic of underlying problems, such as discrimination, inequalities and structural coercion. These attempts reveal attitudes and conceptions towards 'humanity' and the role that technology and technique play in human life. Reflecting the social dimensions of such practice, the ethics of sex selection has to respond to the intricacies of our attempts to reconstruct practice in an ethically meaningful way, so as to be able to identify responsibilities and causality patterns. In effect, a cultural perspective can challenge the appropriateness and sufficiency of the concept of 'choice' and the postulate of freedom of individual choices in ethics. Alternatively, we can argue for a 'third way', between individual determination and coercion from powers in society or family. Thus, we can reflect about 'sex selection' in its relation to the overall desiderate of a 'good life', pondering the meaning and impact of such a practice on the lives of the people affected. Whose good does it concern or express? In the terms of philosophy, such an approach accounts for the process-character of *autonomy* proper ('Autonomie'), as it should be represented in communicative situations, such as in the request for 'informed consent' (Manson & O'Neill 2007).

'Slippery slopes'

In an opinion paper published in the *New Scientist*, a London-based philosopher, A. C. Grayling, argues that prenatal sex selection would not raise principal ethical concern. Using a standard procedure of the analytical approach, Grayling identifies the 'slippery slope' as the main objection against such practice. 'The principal argument offered in opposition is the slippery slope: if we allow a couple to choose their baby's sex, soon people will be choosing to have blond Aryan giants with IQs of a million. Slippery-slope arguments are logically fallacious: drinking one cup of tea does not incur the risk that one will thereupon lose control and proceed to drink a thousand cups of tea' (Grayling 2005; Savulescu 1999a; Harris 1997).

While the slippery slope argument certainly is, to some extent, a matter of assessment of consequences and thereby logically tricky, it also can be appreciated that it expresses moral concern which might be reasoned in more convincing terms.[1] However, merits of slippery slope arguments are not necessarily brought about by default. Accordingly, the case of prenatal sex selection serves as an example for an underlying moral concern and ethical reasoning, the rationale of which applies to established prenatal techniques as well as to preimplantation genetic diagnosis (PGD).

A balanced and informed ethical approach appreciates both concern for the plausibility of predicted practical *consequences* and for the ethical meaningfulness of subjective moral views and *interests*. As it is somehow negatively illustrated in the trivialising metaphor of the 'cup of tea', context indeed matters. By virtue of the intrinsically serious concern of strong moral intuitions, the issues at stake cannot be assessed in a casual manner. Instead, they need to be considered within their proper practical context. Otherwise, the discussion from the outset will be barren of psychological (motivation), social (power) and cultural (values and meaning) reflection.

Methodological assessment

When reconstructed as a heuristic notion, the slippery slope functions as a *preparatory* argument that, if duly accounted for, provides guidance for those who explore the moral validity of concerns about sex selection. It should be noted that the methodological merit of the slippery slope argument is that it highlights the reciprocal interconnection between *maxim* and *consequences*, together with the performative ethical tension between those polarities in practice. Rather than being lightly dismissed, it can support the process of interpretation towards a proper rendering of the social and cultural meaning of the enquired practice, without claiming strong normative power in its own right. The case of sex selection in China highlights the requirement of proper methodology in ethics, because it re-emphasises the importance of context, by virtue of the differences in the relevant cultural, social and political circumstances, such as those in the UK.

Grayling is right to point out the impracticality of 'designing' babies, including their sex. 'If ever IVF became cheap and easy, which it is extremely far from being, and was employed to produce just boys in cultures that prefer them, those cultures would soon find the choice self-defeating.'

He holds a pertinent point by stating the adverse impact of collectively one-sided individual choices of sex, the consequences of which reach beyond the scale of the individuals' narrow interests. Indeed, the imbalanced sex ratios of infants in India and China set clear examples for the counter-productiveness of widely applied technologies for sex determination, in terms of society's and national interests. Even if one regards the common acceptance of the principles of population control and family planning in China as an expression of general concern for the public good, the actual impression of this general consideration is limited. In fact, individual persons', families' and communities' choices can differ from or contradict such concern. Notably, the first Chinese Population and Family Law expressly holds the *couples* responsible for proper family planning. It acknowledges the primary importance of private decision-making, which naturally adheres to its own particular interests.

However, when discussing the ethics of choice, there is no point in defending choices that would produce 'blond Aryan giants with IQs of a million', should this option ever become practical, as Grayling suggests. Beyond the issue of risk assessment, it is largely a matter of metaphysical (moral, religious) opinion and taste rather than a subject for ethical debate. The actual definition of preferential traits is always accidental; here, and as related to China, it falls short of serving its polemic purpose, which might otherwise be well taken in a European and Northern American setting.

The serious trouble with 'preference', or the *bias* in a preference, is the downside of it. In the case of sex selection, as a matter of fact *preference of one implies indifference to or discrimination against another*. The ethical rationale of discriminatory or indifferent preferences stretches beyond personal attitudes and opinion, in that it becomes an organising principle of practice. It should then be considered in its meaning, as it permeates through spatial and temporal ramifications, in recognition of the most likely consequences. In the context of moral reflection, this type of preference is an expression of a fundamental political and social interest and, at the same time, a cause or reason for general orientations in policies and practice. When allied with power or force, it has a potential to affect the conditions of life and to infringe upon the freedom of others.

Moreover, in the social and political spheres, the underlying presumption of (an actually) free and rational choice is problematic. Left without further practical elaboration, the assumption of freedom of choice degenerates into dogmatism, with no practical meaning, or apologetics for any event in the highly unjust 'market of opportunities'.

As matters of practice, social, economic, political, moral and technological factors must be regarded with their influence on decision-making. Even in so-called developed democracies of Western Europe, those
factors form pressures which quite efficiently constrain the liberty of
people's choices in procreation. For example, women are constrained in
their liberty to determine the way in which they wish to procreate by a
range of practical demands from their professional life, or from the
availability of institutions or individuals to help them in daycare for
their children. In the case of China, the notorious policies of obligatory
family planning, population control and the spreading of biotechnologies cannot be discounted in their effect on the reality, and thus morality, of choice. They make the structural reason for the contingency of
'choice' or preference.

It matters how we reconstruct the context of 'good', as it may be regarded as either morally significant or insignificant. The semantics of
Grayling's simile of 'drinking one cup of tea' presuppose an understanding of a natural capacity to desire, to unambiguously identify and
satisfy this desire. Here it is as convenient and plausible to make any
choice, as the respective practical content is *morally irrelevant* from the
outset. Whereas the 'cup of tea' is connected with an individual agent,
his or her physical space and emotional comfort, a preference for a
baby of a certain design is a categorically different matter. It embraces
the additional components of practice, which do make moral sense,
ethical deliberation and action morally relevant and difficult in the first
place.

There is a disregard for the influence of the effects of accumulated
micro-practice over time. The agent may indeed eventually end up having drunk the 'thousand cups of tea', which we cannot see or imagine
when we look at an act as an isolated event, lacking continuity in the dimension of time and causal connectivity in society. The actual situation
is further enriched and complicated by the fact that no such choice is
socially outcome-neutral, for it immediately affects others, such as
spouse, family members or the composition of the world of the expected child. What appeals as good and thus preferable depends to a relevant degree upon the social and cultural context over some expansion
of time. We cannot lightly dismiss the slippery slope argument by referring to inadequate analogies, such as that of drinking tea, in a culturally
meaningful discourse. For the factual availability or non-availability of
choices have an impact on the quality of ethical and cultural analysis of
morality no less than the ways we understand these choices as statements in their own right.

Social ramifications

Since the late 1990s, Chinese and international observers have increasingly paid attention to sex selection as an issue in medical ethics and governance. In 2004, Hudson and den Boer published an extensive study on the missing females in India and the People's Republic of China (PRC) (Hudson and den Boer 2004). This study does not expressly address ethical or bioethical issues, but strategic political and social consequences of the gender imbalance in developing countries, with their regional and global impact. However, much of the material is easily accessible and immediately relevant for ethical and cultural scientific scrutiny. This paper makes extensive use of the material prepared in this book. It also draws on my study on bioethics in China, including data and interviews with experts from different backgrounds. The broad approach adopted here does not focus on particular techniques, preferences or individual cases, but rather on the socially meaningful pattern of the practice of gender- or sex-related selection. This includes such phenomena as systematic discrimination against females, male favouritism and paternalism, targeted abortion of females, infanticide and neglect. Apart from focusing on the present biomedical context, links are made between gender preference and Chinese cultural and philosophical traditions.

Chinese accounts

Chinese medical ethicists have addressed these questions. For example, in an international conference in Hamburg, in 1998, two veteran biologists and medical ethicists from Shanghai, Chen Renbiao and Qiu Xiangxing, examined cases of fatally mistreated and neglected baby girls in medical wards. Their discussion culminated in a dramatic conclusion. 'If our clinicians and other medical workers are ignorant of basic medical morals, they very probably fall short of even minimal humanity' (Chen & Qiu 1999).

Chen and Qiu argue that the practice of discrimination based on gender or other congenital peculiarities contradicts a common moral sense. 'If parents are not aware of behavioural guidelines, which are in accordance with the medical moralities accepted by a great majority of the people, it will be almost impossible to achieve the so-called "informed consent" in its real meaning. To have either a healthy baby, a baby affected with a congenital abnormality or a certain kind of genetic disease, is a natural phenomenon, and its fate cannot be determined by the subjective interests of the parents, not even with high-tech medicine.'

The authors interpret the behaviour of selective killing and neglect in terms of deviance of selfish individuals from basic human duties. In their moral statement they proclaim that, 'The moral and legal responsibility of the parents towards their babies should always be realised, no matter what the physical or mental status of the baby is like. Of course, all doctors should offer medical services at the highest possible level of technology, as provided by the latest achievements of medical sciences, and treat all patients equally, with strict obedience to the principles of medical ethics.'

They propose that, in order to respond properly to the present situation in China, 'the education of medical professionals and medical students in modern medical ethics, and its popularisation among the broad masses of the Chinese people, is of top priority' (Chen & Qiu 1999).

One year later, in 1999, at an international symposium in Shanghai, population experts Gao Xiangdong and Xu Yan described the availability of relevant techniques of sex selection in China and the related social and ethical issues, making a robust moral case against its application: 'We strongly oppose sexual selection because it is detrimental to the national future' (Gao & Xu 2002).

Gao and Xu offer a short introduction into the history of the issue and its awareness in China:

> The unbalanced sex ratio at birth in China has been the subject of attention for researchers, the general public, and policymakers of the Chinese government. Many studies have been carried out to investigate the levels, trends, geographic variations, and causes of China's unbalanced sex ratio at birth and the extreme mortality rate among female infants, as well as their relationships with other socio-economic and demographic variables and their implications for society.

In the 1960s and 1970s, the sex ratio at birth in China was balanced between 106 and 107 (number of boys as related to 100 girls). However, it increased rapidly, from 107.7 in 1980 to 113.0 in 1992. According to statistics from developed countries, the normal sex ratio at birth should remain between 105 and 107. Compared with this normal average, the sex ratio at birth in China has shown an abnormally increasing trend, which indicates the problem of 'missing girls' in China.

Anticipating Hudson and den Boer and other studies, Gao and Xu report that, 'Our analysis shows that the sex ratio at birth observed in China is likely to be caused by a strong preference for a son. The popular use of ultrasound scanning, and the collapse of the rural cooperatives and the medical care system at the village level in the 1980s are the direct causes which have resulted in a high sex ratio at birth in favour of males and an extremely high female infant mortality.'

Here, we find a clear account of most of the factors, which later studies have highlighted and reconfirmed as being crucial for an assessment of sex selection as a social practice in China. They are described as composed of cultural, social and technological elements. Namely, a cultural concern for breeding boys, a social crisis due to the disintegration of established infrastructures of healthcare and social security, together with the accessibility of technological inventions, which provide convenient opportunities that allow sex-selective abortion to become a 'silent practice', hidden from public scrutiny but performed widely (Nie 2005).

In a nutshell, Gao and Xu delineate the ethical issues as follows. 'This sex ratio at birth results in serious demographic problems for society, including a surplus of men on the future marriage market, a delayed age crossing-over, (resulting in extended gaps between the generations), and an abnormally unbalanced sex ratio among children and in the whole population. It also indicates the existence of serious social problems, including ongoing discrimination against girls, social conflicts and cultural changes, and women's relatively low status in the family and society' (Gao & Xu 2002).

Cultural and social patterns

The Hudson and den Boer study has provided impressive evidence for the validity of these descriptions and projections. In their book they conclude in a general statement, setting the current practice in a cultural perspective:

> Gender inequality resulting in various forms of offspring sex selection was evidenced throughout much of China's history. ... Economic, political and social reforms in the latter half of the twentieth century combined to produce a culture in which traditional son preference, coupled with declining fertility and politicized family planning policies resulted in increasing resort to female infanticide and sex-selective abortion. It is likely that these practices will persist. (Hudson & den Boer 2004: 186)

In recent years, a growing volume of literature has been published that illuminates the scientific, social and humanitarian depths of this phenomenon. Xinran, in her collected biographical narratives of contemporary female lives, *The Good Women of China*, refutes the Maoist myth of China's women inhabiting 'Heaven's Half' (Ebrey & Ebrey 1991: 326) by submitting a politically sensitive description of systematic abuse of the female as a commodity (Xinran 2003). In her novel, *Throwaway Daughter*, Ye Ting-Xing ascribes her own unwanted birth as a girl to the failure of the *feng-shui* method to determine her sex properly. Without the erroneous statement from a geomanticist, who saw indication for a boy, she would most likely have been aborted early. Having satisfied the would-be parents' expectations towards a pregnancy with a boy, the Master entirely failed to provide the family with a warning on improbability or an alternative scenario to that of killing or neglect, or support after the birth of a girl (Ye 2003). In this narrative, she was subsequently put into one of the notorious orphanages (Human Rights Watch 1996). Folk-religious practices of sex determination, and the creation of options for reproductive decision-making, have been widely established in China prior to the advent of medical technology. It prepared ready grounds and established the rationales and 'culture' for a bias towards *designing the family* in China. The high social value of having a boy, with its practical consequence of a biased attitude against females, is also expressed in the relative amount of care invested in the early weeks of infancy. The outcome can be seen in the infant mortality rates in the first year of life. Depending on the source, between 61 and 88 male deaths occur per that of 100 females, while the naturally expected rate is 130 (Hudson & den Boer 2004: 176). The overall sex ratio is thus composed of active selection and abortion, or killing, of females and the abandonment of care for female infants, on the one hand, plus increased care and attention for the boys on the other.

This practice can be assessed through clusters of relevant factors. First, all authors agree on the existence of a traditional 'philosophical' bias discriminating against 'the female'. This allegedly structural or even cultural bias often refers to the cosmic duality of *yin* and *yang* that maintains the transformation of all being, reinterpreted socially as genderised, or even biologically as sexualised, polarities. The original, value-neutral and abstract notion of *yin* and *yang* (Roetz 2004)[2] expresses the correlative twofold emanation of the forms of the cosmic-energetic *qi*. It eventually became associated with societal concepts, including gender, especially since the Han dynasty (Swann 1932)[3] and, in a response to Buddhist philosophy, during Tang- and Song-dynastic Neo-Confucianism, namely the 'Rationalist School' of Cheng Yi and Zhu Xi, with its strong patriarchal undercurrent (Munro 1988, Munro 1985). Nowadays, the 'strong, dominating and male' quality of *yang* has acquired the social and biological meaning of 'male' in general, whereas the notion of the 'soft, yielding and female' *yin* is taken to represent the 'female' in the social and biological sense as well.

This naturalistic or ontological turn (Paul 1996) has exerted a strong influence on Chinese thinkers, including contemporary bioethicists (Qiu 2000, 2003; Fan 1997). On the other hand, Chinese feminists are criticising the patriarchal bias in Chinese society on the basis of moral common sense, though they regularly fail to point towards the inherent historical and philosophical inconsistencies among these dominant concepts (Nie 2000; Li 1999).

The cosmological bias is in particular applied as an ideological rationale to support patriarchal family structures and social hierarchy. Underneath the propaganda veil of gender equality, the de facto discrimination of 'Heaven's Half' has continued under the rule of Mao Zedong, especially in terms of structural inequity and sexual exploitation, affecting, for instance, the globally unique situation that more female than male suicides are committed each year in China (Phillips, Liu & Zhang 1999; Lee & Klenmann 2000; Dikötter 1998).

Some sociological features involved in the shaping of the circumstances of sex selection are noteworthy. Considering the ethnic aspect, Hudson and den Boer use data from the 1990 census to show that among the Han people, who make up more than 91 per cent of China's population, the ratio at that time was as high as 111.71. In comparison, the 54 other ethnic groups have an average ratio of 107.5, which comes fairly close to the natural standard[4] (Hudson & den Boer 2004: 164, 170, 178f).

Moreover, there appears to be an urban-rural divide, namely owing to the accepted economic value of males, especially as workers in the highly labour-intensive agricultural and related activities (Yuan 1991: 202) and for the more powerful social functions claimed by men (Hudson & den Boer 2004: 155). In short-period economic terms, on the micro-level, having girls can create disadvantages for families; traditionally, there is no expected compensation for the investment in their upbringing, education and the costs for out-marrying (e.g. dowries).

Although here lies an obvious conflict between long- and short-term interests, for many families, preference for boys is plainly based on pragmatic calculation, which may or may not conflict with emotional or social values. Still, after a generation's worth of family planning policies, China is now confronted with an alarming shortage of young brides. Restrictive family-planning policies have resulted in a drastic gender imbalance. It is assumed that 'the country is missing 50 million girls who would have been born if not for sex-based abortions and female infanticide. Sons are valued far more than daughters in China because males maintain the family line and care for parents when they grow old. Girls, on the other hand, leave their parents' home for their husband's clan when they marry,' as *Time Magazine* describes it (Beech 2002).

Various factors stand out as important in the practice of gender selection. First, the economic conditions of the communities have a significant influence on the procreative decision-making of couples. It appears that the most competitive regions in a state of dynamic transformation show high sex ratios. Gu Baochang and Xu Yi have observed gender ratios at opposite poles in terms of developmental scale. They have either been socio-economically advanced for a long time, with modern attitudes towards gender, or they are so economically and socially backward that the state shows some leniency (Gu & Xu 1994: 423).

A second factor relevant to gender preference is birth order. Hudson and den Boer show that birth order plays a role in the readiness of parents to consider the options of sex-selective abortion or even to abandon their child:

> The typical profile of an abandoned child is a healthy newborn girl who has one or more older sisters and no brothers. She is abandoned because her birth parents already have daughters and want a son. These birth parents routinely say that they did not want to abandon the child but that, given their desire for a son, birth planning policies left them 'no choice'. (Hudson & den Boer 2004: 170)

Hudson and den Boer provide convincing evidence for their claim that, in China, 'as in India, gender bias does not come into play strongly with the first child, despite the one-child policy. With the first child, most parents are willing to avoid sex selection' (Hudson & den Boer 2004: 164). Given the efforts required for organising a birth-order scheme in practice, this observation suggests that Chinese families genuinely hesitate to consider abandoning a child. Thus, evidence contradicts the notion of a strongly discriminatory attitude against females in China on justifiable cultural grounds.

A third factor influential in the occurrence of sex selection is the role of the level of education of the mothers. The ratio among children from women with a diploma from higher education is, at 110.7, significantly lower (albeit still relatively high) than that of women with junior high school education, who have 116.2 boys per 100 girls.[5] These data suggest a correlation between academic, social and related economic status and hesitation to opt against having a girl (Hudson & den Boer 2004: 179).

An inherited bias

Most of the elements of contemporary practice of selective abortion and infanticide can be found throughout China's history, together with its criticism and state action undertaken against it. In late Imperial China, 'the Chinese apparently regarded infanticide as a form of postnatal abortion through which they could choose the number, spacing, and sex of their children in response to short-term economic conditions as well as their long-term family-planning goals' (Lee, Campbell & Tan 1992: 146).

However, 'infanticide has in fact been constantly condemned throughout Chinese history. Numerous exhortative books and tracts have been published as moral correctives and various penalties ... have been imposed by successive dynasties' (Hudson & den Boer 2004: 141). During the Song, Yuan and Ming dynasties, for example, infanticide was made a serious crime. Incentives were introduced for families to raise more than two girls. A prominent argument was that 'the crime of infanticide was in defiance of nature itself' (T'ein 1988: 28-30). The tragedy of the situation at that time may be inferred from the symbol of the famous sixteenth-century stone of Fuzhou, which stated: 'Girls may not be drowned here' (Jimmerson 1990: 50).

The legalist philosopher, Han Fei, refers to the 'convenience' of infanticide, as an argument against the innate goodness of human nature, which was propagated by the Confucian mainstream:

> The relation of parents to their children is such that they congratulate each other if a son is born, but they (may) kill a daughter. The children equally come out of the parental womb. The reason that one congratulates on a son, but kills a daughter, is that parents merely consider their future conveniences and calculate their long-term benefit. Thus even parents in relation to their children use a calculating mind. How much more holds this true (for politics) where there is no parental kindness.[6] (Roetz 1993: 258)

This Machiavellian rationale betrays an awareness of a moral sense and disillusion towards the practicality of a policy of altruistic humanism. Han Fei's profound and prudent suspicion against the human capacity for genuine moral interests cannot invalidate the conflicting sense of moral discomfort on his part, which has lead most moral philosophers, and Confucians in particular, to a contradictory conclusion, namely to cultivate the families and the state (Döring 2003a).

Technology in the political box

Notwithstanding the importance of social and cultural influences on attitudes towards gender and sex, a crucial cause for the change in sex-selective practice in contemporary China obviously lies in the availability of medical technology, under the circumstances of a restrictive population policy. Empirical studies have unanimously proven that the ratio began to increase significantly at the very time when ultrasound devices were introduced for common clinical use, in the late 1970s. Gu and Xu state that 'the areas with high birth ratios are also areas with the greatest popularity of ultrasound equipment' (Gu & Xu 1994: 426). After a continuing decrease in the sex ratio since 1936 (calculated at 114), almost down to 106 in 1965, the 'Cultural Revolution' terminated this trend and reversed it, with a slow increase towards 108 in 1972. In the period since 1984, the curve is suddenly peaking, once more reaching the level of 1936, a ratio of 114, approaching that of 1990 (Hudson & den Boer 2004: 151).

Owing to the availability of ultrasound and other prenatal diagnostic or fertility techniques (sperm-sorting, IVF), Chinese couples under pressure to consider abandoning a child are now more often able to interfere at an earlier stage of gestation, by aborting the embryo or foetus. Hence, the more recent statistics of ratios at birth might come closer in accuracy to the actual ratio of surviving infants,[7] since the impact of postnatal killing (i.e. by neglect) had declined. A similar impact on the gender ratio of the availability of sex-screening technology has been described for Taiwan. In the absence of a strict population control policy in Taiwan, and with the more educated use of contraceptives, Taiwan does not account for a relevant practice of infanticide or neglect; the ratio, though unnaturally high, remains relatively low compared to the mainland (Freedman, Chang & Sun 1994).[8]

The significance of prenatal diagnostic technology has been discussed predominantly in literature regarding eugenics and the abuse of women in China (Dikötter 1998; Döring 1998a) but less attention has been paid to the social meaning and cultural implications of sex selection. Among the cultural elements that make it difficult to profile Chinese attitudes and concepts towards the social and moral sense of an early human life, there is the fuzzy concept of the meaning of 'birth' (Stafford 1995) and of the beginning of the full moral status of human life. Although the moment of birth is formally significant as a reference point for administration and civil legislation, it does not necessarily bear more than technical meaning in cultural and moral terms. Common sense has it that a newborn child is counted as 'age of one' (yi sui), suggesting that it had been 'socially born' to the family earlier. Even libertarian bioethicists in China accept that the human embryo has some innate value by virtue of being a human life; hence they discourage late abortions and propagate a gradualist conceptualisation of becoming a 'full' human being (Qiu 2000; Döring 2003b; Lee 2002). On the other hand, unwanted infants are frequently killed some time after birth. Given the fuzzy concept and poor moral significance of the incidence of birth, which does not suffice to protect infants from maltreatment, there appears to be a grey moral zone, leaving the moral meaning and status of early human lives in flux.

It is unclear at which stage of early human development the selection of genetic or gender traits does or ought to become an issue. The premature level and controversial character of the related debates on the moral status of an embryo, foetus and newborn implies that the increased level of attention to this area of life is rather recent (Döring 2003b; 2004). Public discourse and awareness is required for framing and assessing the prenatal gender issues related to sex selection (Nie 2005). Obviously, people are concerned about the killing and neglect of infants. However, the same moral reasoning that applies to the protection and esteem of infants and the rejection of late abortions will make it more difficult to justify selective abortion of viable foetuses, even at an earlier stage of development.

Considering the hesitation of Chinese couples to abandon a child of the 'wrong sex', it is conceivable that the particular societal and cultural biases toward gender are changing. Biases might be transforming into less harmful preferences, such as family balancing. Indeed, sociological findings support a general inclination towards the model of a balanced nuclear family, including at least one girl and one boy.[9] Examples of mistreatment of young girls seem to be exceptions rather than conforming to widely accepted cultural standards.

Policy responses: regulation

As Li Xiaorong has remarked, in her standard work, Licence to Coerce, the Chinese government has generally failed to carry out punishment for female infanticide in the past (Li 1996: 163). This accounts for the discrepancy between state policy and legislation vis-à-vis its implementation in China. In 1983, China's Central Propaganda Department called for 'the protection of infant girls, and also of women who have given birth to daughters, from social ostracism and physical cruelty' (Yuan 1991: 131). In 2000, The White Paper on Population and Development, released by the State Council of the PRC, did not mention sex-selective abortions, though it addressed the mistreatment of girls (Hudson & den Boer 2004: 174).

Despite the difficulties in implementing legislation, the state has criticised and periodically sanctioned infanticide, reflecting that it was commonly and continuously regarded as a serious issue. The regulatory impact of legislation on the practice of sex selection is apparent though not satisfying. For example, after the introduction of the legal prohibition of sex determination, the protection of female infants and the policy of licensing second birth allowances for couples who have borne a handicapped or a female child, the adverse effects of social and economic pressures on the family shifted from the first child to the second or third one.

It can be expected that the systematic building of a legal state and the associated culture of law, with a reliable and independent function to protect the interests of the vulnerable populations in particular, together with significantly improved health insurance and social security systems, would prompt greater compliance (Döring 2003c).

Sex selection has been an explicit public issue in China since 1993, when government and Party distributed it through the leading mass media and put it onto the agenda of state-funded research. Various legal actions have been undertaken:

- The disputed 'Mothers and Infants Health Care Law' of 1995, in Article 32, stipulates that 'Sex identification of a foetus by technical means shall be strictly forbidden, except when it is positively needed in medical terms' (Döring 1998b). This stipulation is reconfirmed in the 'Amended Guidelines on Human Reproduction Technology and Sperm Banks', as of July 2003, (under the header of the ethical principle of the common good). These clauses emphasise that it is against professional ethics and the law for medical researchers and physicians to perform sex-determining diagnosis.
- The 'Population and Family Planning Law' of 2002 states in Article 22, 'Discrimination against and mistreatment of women who give birth to female children or who suffer from infertility are prohibited. Discrimination against mistreatment and abandonment of female infants are prohibited.'
- The 'Marriage Law' of 2002, in Article 21, prescribes that 'infant drowning, deserting and any other acts causing serious harm to infants and infanticide shall be prohibited.'

Similar statements, referring to gender equality, non-discrimination and a duty to care, are expressed in the Chinese constitution and Chinese Communist Party communications. The Chinese government is clearly aware of the international attention paid to these issues. In a white paper disseminated through the website of the Permanent Mission of the PRC to the United Nations, it claims:

> The Chinese government and the society as a whole have paid close attention to the recent tendency of the high sex ratio. The problem will be gradually solved through heightened publicity and education, and measures have been taken to guarantee the legal rights and interests of women and children; to severely prohibit, except when called for medically, the technical examination of a foetus for determining sex followed by selective abortion; and to improve birth report and statistical systems.[10]

The official website of *Xinhuanet* reported in 2003 that 'new regulations in southern Guangdong Province echo the prohibition of identifying a foetus' gender and selective artificial pregnancy without proper medical need, which is distinctly defined in the state law. Guangdong regulations specify that people who induce abortion without official approval will not be permitted to reproduce again, effectively curbing abortions just because parents want a boy' (Xinhuanet 2003).

In January 2003, 'Regulations on the Prohibition of the Identification of the Sex of a Foetus with no Medical Purpose and Abortions Based on Gender Preferences' came into effect. Therein, in particular, Article 3 states that 'any identification of the sex of a foetus with no medical purpose and abortions based on gender preferences are strictly prohibited.'

Professional and legal oversight are clearly regulated and defined here. Regulatory procedures for monitoring exceptional cases of medically indicated sex determination are laid out in detail, according to the different levels of jurisdiction and administration. The same applies to abortions. Medical personnel are obliged to explore the social background of the family and rule out sex selection as the reason for an abortion. Pregnancies are to be registered and monitored systematically.

Although these regulations can raise concerns about the freedom and privacy of pregnant women, they quite clearly express a serious dedication on the side of the state to contain the practice of sex selection in China, and make oversight more effective.

Discussion

What does the situation of sex selection in China tell us about the preferences of Chinese parents? What are the actual choices they make when they decide to selectively abort or abandon a female? How can the ambiguity in the attitudes towards born and unborn children be mended so as to encourage a consistent practice? How would couples decide and reason under conditions of greater freedom and/or economic advancement? The desired public debate would make efforts to integrate the conflicting rationales of acceptance of abortion versus the moral repugnance towards infanticide and abandonment.

In China, assessment of sex selection is, in most cases, framed in relation to harm, rather than as a discourse on rights. The concept of having a right to procreate, although it is enshrined in the national legislation, is not widely appreciated in China. The language of the debates focuses on duties or obligations and tends to understand rights as functions of these. The principal obligation in this context is to avoid harm to members of society or the relevant community, and to increase the benefit of one's own family, over generations.

As long as attention must be paid to the abandoning and killing of infants, it is unlikely that the protection and non-discrimination of prenatal beings will be assessed in other than primarily prudential or utilitarian terms. The focus of the moral pressures towards reform highlights the general gender situation in China. As Hudson and den Boer describe it, 'Women have gained the ability to control their own money and choose their occupations. With regard to choices concerning their own bodies, however, women lost control over family planning in the late 1970s' (Hudson & den Boer 2004: 150). Here, it is not only the state that interferes; the family and the community have a strong stake in controlling family planning. Procreation is an area in society where females are discriminated against and disadvantaged, as they are expected to reproduce according to the requirements of state regulation, while being held accountable for the outcome by family and community. Besides their political and moral seriousness, the recent legislation still should be reviewed in consideration of a paternalistic attitude by the state, the party and medical ethicists. They do not always take into account pressures on pregnant women and their spouses. In short, sex selection in China cannot be adequately assessed in terms of positive preferences and choices. One major reason is the joint impact of population policy, biotechnology and the liberal market on reproductive decision-making.

The example of sex selection in China illustrates the importance of cultural and social context in the assessment of ethical practice, as the rationale of the slippery slope argument commends it. Grayling's claim that disregarding societal background, if sex selection were 'employed to produce just boys in cultures that prefer them, those cultures would soon find the choice self-defeating', may be sound in some contexts but is not in others. In order to be implemented, the effective rejection of sex selection requires political initiative from the state, namely legislation and implementation. Only within an existing robust societal constitution, with its supporting institutional infrastructure, one free from undue pressures and one which prevents individual cases of abuse, can 'choosing the sex' be considered as an option for citizens. The 'slippery slope' will have fulfilled its purpose and can be dismissed, in the event that the established normative structures actively repel the excessive practice of instrumental sex selection, when social and moral structures prevail that will not likely accumulate towards massive moral or social troubles and individual tragedy. As far as China and many other countries are concerned, the reality is a far cry from such a state.

Moreover, China's unbalanced sex ratio amplifies the effects of accumulation of individual practices that are basically not concerned with the aggregate. Accordingly, the prognosis that 'cultures find it self-defeating' is pointless, because cultures are not acting subjects.

The discussion above has also demonstrated that ethics refers to the practical quality of action, as it can be encountered in the maxims of an agent, that is, higher-order purposes that organise one's will, preceding considerations about consequences. For example, 'sex selection' is not a plausible maxim, but, for example, 'achieving better living conditions', or 'preventing one's kin from harm', can be. A genuinely ethical reason to go beyond the realm of the slope is not that it is logically faulty, but that it is limited to social and political matters. An investigation into medical ethics should connect the relevant psychological (motivation), social (power) and cultural (values and meaning) patterns of a given practice, so that they may instigate an understanding of the structure of practice.

Moreover, this analytical approach, with its off-hand rejection of the slippery slope argument, fails to appreciate the central theme of the debate of the ethics of technology. There is no particular ethical merit in discussing certain techniques (other than indirectly via risks and benefits), because they are endowed with moral meaning solely through practice. An ethical assessment can best take place through a hermeneutic method, such as performed above, exploring and reconstructing individual cases within their respective contexts. This approach addresses the relational interplay between individual determination and coercion from powers in society or family. It indicates that the practices shall be observed in perspective, according to their relative position in a process of cultivation, that is, within a scenario of hope.

In short, in contemporary China, it would be utterly inappropriate to assess the issues of sex selection in terms of 'freedom of choice' or as an 'individual's right to independent procreative decision-making'. As Adorno has expressed it, there is no 'Right Way within Wrongness'.[11] Any attempt to declare the de facto practice in China on face value as an expression of individual, social or cultural self-determination would be unsympathetic and support political and social apologetics. It would even fall behind the prudential insight of the Communist Party and Government, who clearly indicate the need to interfere and build civil capacities. Whereas we cannot get much advice from China about proper sex selection, discussion of the Chinese situation re-emphasises the pertinent ethical perspective.

Notes

* This is a modified version of a paper entitled, 'What's in a choice? Ethical, Cultural and Social Dimensions of Sex Selection in China', published in HUMONTOGENET 2(1), 2008: 11-24; doi 10.1002/huon.200800002, on 17 April 2008 (http://www3.interscience.wiley.com/cgi-bin/fulltext/118638826/PDFSTART?CRETRY=1&SRETRY=0).

1   Such an effect is quite often found in the process of moral arguments under ethical scrutiny. Another example is the relevance of 'repugnance' as an indicator for potential ethical wrong (deCastro 2002).

2   Accordingly, *Xunzi* says, 'When heaven and earth work together, the myriad things are brought into existence. When yin and yang get in contact with each other, transformation and change begin. When human nature and artifice (*wei*) work together, the world gets into order (*zhi*). Heaven (nature) can produce the things, but it cannot give them a differentiated structure (*bian*). Earth can bear man, but it cannot bring him order (*zhi*). All things in the universe as well as man and similar beings depend on the sage for getting their proper position (*fen*).' *Xunzi* 19, cf. also *Xunzi* 9. Likewise, Mengzi rejects the notion of the normativity of *yin* and *yang* (*Mengzi* 2 A 2) (Roetz 2004).

3   The famous example of a model female Confucian is depicted in Swann (1932: 82-90).

4   Inconsistencies in the quoted ratios are due to methodological and statistical deviations. However, they do not affect the validity of the general trend and proportionality as it matters here.

5   When analysing the relevant statistical data, it should be noted that in many cases they refer to infants who survived the first year of life rather than newborns (Hudson & den Boer 2004: 151).

6   It is interesting to note that Hudson and den Boer omit the last two sentences, which formulate the lesson of this case, according to Han Fei. Thereby, quote and translation fail to account for the sense of intrinsic conflict between family morality and raison d'etat that is the essence of this passage (Hudson and den Boer 2004: 139).

7   'Sex ratios are more indicative of surviving infants' sex ratios than of sex ratios at birth. ... (Female infants) die soon after birth as a result of deliberate action by parents or through neglect to the point of fatal illness' (Hudson & den Boer 2004: 151).

8   Due to screening technology, in Taiwan the sex ratio began to rise from 106.6 in 1985 to 109.5 in 2000. In 1990, the sex ratio in Taiwan was 110.2, whereas in the PRC it reached 114.7 (Gu & Roy 1995; Hudson & den Boer 2004: 57f).

9   The UN's Household, Gender, and Age Project reports that the percentage of nuclear families increased steadily since 1949, while the percentage of lineal and joint families dropped slowly (United Nations University 1993). In a report issued by the Information Office of the State Council Of the People's Republic of China, dated August 1995, distributed under the title 'Family Planning in China' and dated 28 December 2004, it says that the 'nuclear family is becoming the major form of modern Chinese families' (www. china-un.ch/eng/bjzl/t176938.htm).

10 www.china-un.ch/eng/bjzl/t176938.htm, Internet Website of the Permanent Mission of PRC to the UN in Switzerland, download 21 January 2005.

11 The common translation is: 'Wrong life cannot be lived rightly' (Adorno 1951).

11 Genetic Testing and Diet-related Disease in Asia: Preventing Diseases or Misleading Marketing?

Helen Wallace

Introduction

Major social and economic shifts in agriculture and diet have led to an intense debate about the future of food and a tension between what Lang and Heasman (2004) describe as the 'Life Sciences Integrated Paradigm' – reliant on the industrial-scale application of biotechnology – and the 'Ecologically Integrated Paradigm' – with a focus on dietary diversity and organic foods. Advocates of the 'Life Sciences Integrated Paradigm' commonly claim that diet-related diseases, particularly the current global epidemic of obesity and associated type 2 diabetes, can be fixed technically, by a combination of individual health screening and new food products ('functional foods'), known as 'personalised nutrition'. In this scenario, individualised testing for disease risk is often assumed to be based on screening for common genetic variants, perhaps combined with other biological markers of disease risk (collectively known as 'biomarkers').

Food is an important aspect of human well-being, not only an instrument to achieve health (Görman 2006). Görman characterises the main ethical issues for personalised nutrition as:

- Autonomy: The rights and integrity of each individual should be supported in connection with the use of personalised nutrition.
- Beneficence: Personalised nutrition should be used in order to contribute to a good life in line with the values of each person involved.
- Non-maleficence: Personalised nutrition should be used so as to avoid or minimise harm.
- Justice: The benefits of personalised nutrition should be fairly distributed.

He recommends that genetic testing should be based on solid knowledge; screening should only be used when clearly beneficial; specially trained persons should collect information from genetic tests and carry through counselling on a personal basis; and marketing of genetic tests sold directly to the public should be discouraged. Görman also warns that, although development of special products for personalised nutrition may be necessary in some cases, this may lead to a medicalisation of diet.

Although important, this ethical analysis does not consider the broader political context which is likely to determine whether these safeguards are implemented in practice. An increasingly pervasive genetic worldview and expectations about new genetic technologies in the future are profoundly shaping conceptions of health and illness (Petersen 2006). Several interacting processes have led to the 'biomedicalisation' of health in the US, involving: major political economic shifts; a new focus on health and risk and surveillance biomedicines; the 'technoscientisation' of biomedicine; transformations of the production, distribution, and consumption of biomedical knowledge; and transformations of bodies and identities (Clarke et al 2003). These developments are taking place within the context of a strong, and increasingly globalised, commitment to a new 'knowledge-based economy', in which genetic information and biotechnologies are seen as playing a key part. In the US and Europe, tensions between the demand to stimulate innovation and the need to protect consumers have led to a situation where, in general, regulatory agencies do not have the statutory authority to assess the clinical validity or utility of most genetic tests, or their social, legal or ethical implications – despite a consensus view in advisory reports that genetic tests should not enter routine clinical practice without independent evaluation (Hogarth et al 2007).

Asia is at the forefront of the global epidemic of diet-related disease, is a potentially large market for predictive genetic tests and associated products, and has a number of research institutes involved in this type of research. There is a strong political commitment to move towards 'knowledge-based' economies, albeit with very different stages of implementation in different countries (Asian Development Bank 2007).

This chapter discusses whether personalised nutrition is a good research priority for health in Asia and whether health claims for genetic tests are likely to be adequately regulated.

Chronic diet-related disease in Asia

Chronic diet-related diseases – such as type 2 diabetes – are a major, growing threat to global health. The World Health Organization (WHO) now refers to a global 'epidemic' of obesity and has warned that many countries are suffering a 'double burden' of both undernutrition and obesity. In 2004, the WHO predicted that, of the 35 million people expected to die in 2005 from heart disease, stroke, cancer and other chronic diseases, only about 20 per cent would be in high-income countries. Lack of food, famine and malnutrition are still the biggest problems for poor people in the poorest countries. However, in most middle-income countries the poorest people are now those at the *highest* risk of obesity and chronic diseases, such as heart disease and diabetes (Popkin & Gordon-Larsen 2004). An estimated 80 per cent of heart disease, stroke and type 2 diabetes, and 40 per cent of cancer could be avoided through healthy diets, regular physical activity and avoidance of tobacco use (Epping-Jordan et al 2005). For example, a large-scale study in China considerably reduced the incidence of type 2 diabetes using a combination of improved diets and physical activity (Schatz & Pfohl 2001).

Major modifications in diet have taken place worldwide since the second half of the twentieth century, beginning in industrial countries, followed more recently by developing countries (World Health Organization 2003). Traditional plant-based diets have been rapidly replaced by high-fat energy-dense diets with a substantial content of animal foods. At the same time there has been a decrease in levels of physical activity. Per capita food consumption has increased more rapidly in East Asia than in any other region. The increase in dietary fat supply has also been particularly rapid in East Asia, and China has experienced the biggest shift. There are now an estimated 40 million diabetics in China, increasing at a rate of 1.2 million a year, and an estimated 200-300 million people are overweight, with over 70 million obese (Zheng et al 2004). Obesity rates in children are 8.1 per cent in urban areas and 3.1 per cent in rural ones (Anon 2006). The 'nutrition transition' is a global problem, and many Asian countries are at the forefront of these rapid changes. However, impact does differ from one country to another: for example, the Republic of Korea modernised earlier than most Asian countries, but has successfully retained elements of the traditional diet so that the rate of increase in fat intake has been relatively low (Kim et al 2001).

Personalised nutrition and the 'genetic revolution'

A genetic revolution in health has been widely predicted in which genetic tests will be used to identify those individuals who are genetically susceptible to common diseases, such as heart disease and cancer. Some geneticists envisage a future in which individuals take a battery of genetic tests, at birth or later in life, to determine their individual 'genetic susceptibility' or predisposition to disease (Collins 1999; Sander 2000; Bell 1998). In theory, once the risk of particular combinations of genotype and environmental exposure is known, medical interventions (including lifestyle advice, screening or medication) can then be targeted at 'high-risk' groups or individuals, with the aim of preventing disease (Collins & McKusick 2001).

However, this approach to health is controversial. Concerns include the shift in the level of analysis from the population to the individual, leading to the neglect of social and economic factors (Pearce 1996; Food Ethics Council 2005); the 'geneticisation' of health and illness and its potential wider implications, including surveillance and control (Petersen 1998); the oversimplification of the role of genes and environment in common diseases (Baird 2001); the limitations of this strategy for improving health (Vineis et al 2005); and the role of commercial influences on the research agenda (Baird 2002).

A wide range of companies is expected to play a role in personalised nutrition, as a means of adding value to the food supply chain. These include:
- biotechnology companies, which plan to undertake gene-based testing of consumers;
- processed food and supplement companies, which will formulate new products and test and manufacture them;
- food and feed ingredients companies, which will produce new 'value-added' food ingredients;
- food processing companies, which will process foodstuffs to concentrate or extract desirable food components;
- agricultural biotechnology companies, which will apply genomics and genetics to crops and meat-producing animals to increase components with human health value.

The focus of commercial interest in nutritional genomics (nutrigenomics) is in achieving two overlapping aims: developing new functional foods which can be marketed as providing health benefits (or 'optimising well-being') for consumers; and individualising diet – tailoring diets to each individual's 'unique biochemical needs' using genetic tests and perhaps other types of tests (ILSI 2002). This strategy is being driven by two factors: firstly, the need for growth in a competitive market, and secondly, the desire to neutralise concern about the epidemic of obesity and avoid government-imposed public health protection measures (such as bans on advertising unhealthy products, or limits on the salt and sugar content of processed foods).

Genetic medicine is expected to create a new class of 'unpatients', who are not ill but who are treated for their *risk* of future illness. Jonsen et al (1996) conclude that the prognostic unknowns and complexities raise the primary ethical implication for the clinical transaction, namely, what constitutes truthful, accurate genetic information for the 'unpatient'.

Recent ethical concerns in the US and Europe have focused on direct-to-consumer sales of unregulated genetic tests (Gollust et al 2002; American College of Medical Genetics 2004; Haga et al 2003; Vineis & Christani 2004; Humphries et al 2004; Wallace 2005a). Few genetic susceptibility tests are clinically valid or useful and many companies have made misleading claims. Many of these tests are combined with dietary advice and recommendations to take supplements.

The food industry has now begun investing in some of these genetic testing companies as a means to market 'genetically tailored' products (Wallace 2006a, b). It sees 'functional foods' (foods marketed at a premium to 'optimise' health) as a new area for growth, and genetic testing as a future marketing tool. Nutrigenomics and personalised nutrition are being widely promoted as a solution to diet-related disease (Kaput et al 2005).

Nutrigenomics and nutrigenetics in Asia

In its simplest form, nutrigenomics is based on the idea that diet should be tailored to an individual's genetic make-up or genotype (this is sometimes called nutrigenetics). Nutrigenomics research may also include other biological measurements (not just a person's genotype, but also measurements of gene expression or metabolism). In the future, some of these other measurements (collectively known as 'biomarkers') may also be used to 'personalise' nutrition or to help design new functional foods.

The food industry's research group, the International Life Sciences Institute (ILSI), is heavily involved in nutrigenomics research and sees Asia as a potential market for personalised nutrition. ILSI Japan coordinates a nutrigenomics research group at the University of Tokyo (27 companies are involved), and ILSI South East Asia's '1st International Conference on Nutrigenomics – Opportunities in Asia' was held in Singapore in December 2005, and involved scientists from Thailand, Indonesia, China, Korea, India and Japan.

China is the only developing country in the world to have participated in the international Human Genome Project (HGP) and ranks fourth in the world in genome sequencing capability (Anon 2001). China's Institute of Nutritional Sciences, established in Shanghai in November 2003, is one of several institutes in Asia now undertaking nutrigenomic research.

The global food retail market is worth US $ 3,500 billion (IGD 2005). The US is the biggest market but sales in China are growing the fastest. To the food industry, nutrigenomics provides an opportunity to design new products, attempt new 'personalised' marketing strategies (based on genetic test results, or other types of tests) and to claim that it is responding to public concern about the growing epidemic of diet-related disease. The aim is to 'prevent disease and improve quality of life through functional foods and tailored diets' (Institute of Food Technologists, undated). However, the business model relies on 'patent protected, value-added products' commanding a premium price (Mehrotra 2004).

Modern functional food research began in Japan, with a large-scale government-funded research project beginning in 1984. More than 200 functional food products (including soft drinks, yoghurts, biscuits, cookies, sugar, candy, pudding, tofu, vinegar, chocolate and powdered soup) had been approved under the Japanese Food for Specified Health Use (FOSHU) regulations by May 2001 (Arai 2002). In China, many traditional Chinese medicines (such as ginseng, gingko leaf and royal jelly) may be regarded as traditional functional foods and are legally approved by the Ministry of Public Health (Peverelli 2001). However, marketing trends also mean that many new functional food products are being sold in China, including some imported ones (Anon 2005).

Genetic tests combined with nutritional advice or dietary supplements are already being marketed directly to consumers, largely in the US (Wallace 2006a). These tests have been widely criticised by geneticists for being potentially misleading (Vineis & Christani 2004; Humphries et al 2004). However, the marketing of this type of test is likely to increase and spread to other countries.

For example, Sciona, originally a UK company, was forced to withdraw genetic tests combined with dietary advice from the British high street retailers in 2001, following criticism from leading scientists. It relocated to the US, obtained new investment from the major food ingredients companies DSM and BASF, and relaunched its product. Sciona was one of the companies subjected to an investigation by the United States Government Accountability Office (USGAO) in 2006. The investigation concluded that its tests mislead people by making predictions that are medically unproven, and that the test results may needlessly alarm consumers into thinking that they need to buy a costly supplement in order to prevent an illness (USGAO 2006). The company is already exploring the Asian Pacific market and recently partnered with an Australian laboratory to pursue its Asian business further (Halliday 2007).

In 2005, the Japanese company Ci:Labo launched a home obesity gene testing service (Anon 2005), although no validated genetic susceptibility tests for obesity then existed.

Limitations of personalised nutrition

The advocates of personalised nutrition claim that as well as delaying the onset of disease, it could optimise and maintain human health (Clemens & Pressman 2004). However, personalised nutrition could also harm health by targeting the wrong dietary advice at the wrong people and confusing healthy-eating messages.

The two main concerns are: (1) genetic tests and functional foods are targeted at the relatively wealthy and do nothing to help lower socio-economic groups or people in poorer countries; and (2) biology is complex, which makes individual risks inevitably uncertain and hard to predict, and limits the usefulness of targeting lifestyle advice at 'high-risk' individuals.

Rather than increasing the availability of existing healthy products (such as vegetables), or making regulated reductions in the levels of salt, sugar and saturated fats in processed foods, personalised nutrition means designing new 'value-added' products and marketing them as tailored to an individual's personal risk of future illness. Genetic tests and functional foods are targeted at richer consumers (sometimes called the 'worried well'), who can afford the extra cost. This does nothing to help lower socio-economic groups who are more likely to be the victims of fat dumping, 'food deserts' and segregated marketing: the mass marketing to lower socio-economic groups of cheaper, processed products high in fat and sugar. Nor does it tackle the 'politics of food' and issues such as agricultural subsidies, which ensure overproduction of unhealthy food ingredients (Nestle 2002).

Although genetic testing combined with dietary advice has been widely promoted as a means to tackle common diet-related diseases, few genes have been identified which could be used reliably in this way (Joost et al 2007). For example, the recently discovered FTO gene is the first common genetic obesity susceptibility gene to have been confirmed in multiple data sets (Frayling et al 2007), despite numerous previous published claims to have identified such genes (Barsch et al 2000; Rosmond 2003). However, the FTO gene accounts for only about 1 per cent of the variance in body mass index (BMI) in the UK. Furthermore, a recently published study by the Institute of Nutritional Sciences in China found that variants in this gene are not associated with obesity in a Chinese Han population (Li et al 2007). Similarly, newly discovered genetic variants linked with type 2 diabetes do not provide sufficient diagnostic accuracy, either alone or in combination, to be clinically useful (Weedon et al 2006; Zeggini & McCarthy 2007) and the body's response to dietary fats and salt intake is highly complex and appears to involve multiple genes and biological pathways, each of small effect (Masson et al 2002; Masson & McNeill 2005; Liu et al 2004).

Existing tests for common genetic variants that are already being marketed, largely in the US but also globally via the Internet, have been widely criticised by scientists as misleading consumers. Although new discoveries may improve the clinical value of such tests, claims for a future of personalised nutrition tend to ignore the increasing scientific recognition of biological complexity, which makes individual risks inevitably uncertain and hard to predict.

Overall, the scientific evidence for the role of genes in susceptibility to obesity, type 2 diabetes, heart disease, cancer, allergies, osteoporosis and neurological disorders is weak and contradictory, except in a few special cases (Wallace 2006a, b). Claims for a high 'heritability' of common diseases rest on outdated assumptions: for example, that interactions between multiple genes and metabolic pathways do not play a significant role in the development of these conditions (Wallace 2006c). Genes do play an important role in the body's cells and how they respond to diet, and gene-diet interactions do appear to exist at the level of individual genes and nutrients. In most cases, though, genetic differences appear to make only small and subtle differences to a person's risk of diet-related disease and hence very little difference to the foods they should eat. Diets contain multiple foods, foods contain multiple nutrients and the body digests these nutrients through multiple biological pathways, involving many different genes and other factors.

Even if people can be informed of their genetic risk correctly, and they take the advice they are given, targeting the people with high-risk genes may not be good for public health. There are three main reasons for this:

1. *Targeting the high-risk group is often much less effective than changing the diet of the whole population.* Unless the bad health effects of a high-risk diet occur only in the people with high-risk genes, there will be people with low-risk genes who also get the diet-related disease. In many cases, *more* people in this group will get the disease, because there will usually be more people in it. In situations like this, most cases of disease will be missed by targeting dietary advice at the people at high genetic risk (Vineis et al 2005).

2. *The people who have most to gain by changing diets may not be the same as those who are at the highest genetic risk.* This depends on whether the reduction in risk that can be achieved by changing diets is larger for the people at high genetic risk than the people at low genetic risk. If it is, there is said to be a 'gene-diet interaction'.

However, there is no consensus on the magnitude of gene-diet interactions, except for the major food intolerances (to milk, fava beans and alcohol), and complex interactions may prove impossible to quantify (Taioli & Garte 2002).

3. *Deciding whom to target may be difficult if the dietary factor being studied causes more than one disease.* Unhealthy diets can cause many different diseases (for example, eating large amounts of sugary foods can increase the risk of dental caries, type 2 diabetes and obesity, and the latter increases the risk of other diseases, such as some cancers). It is possible (even likely) that people who are more susceptible to some of these diseases will be less susceptible to others. For example, a diet based on 'junk foods' high in fat, sugar and salt will increase the risk of most of the 'big killer' diseases. This means that more genetic research is unlikely to change the basic message – everyone should try to avoid eating too much of these foods, whatever genes they may have.

Personalised nutrition also raises broader social implications. Concerns include: how personal genetic data will be stored and used, including for research or 'direct marketing' of products; whether the police or governments will be given access to commercial genetic databases (Kaye 2006); and whether people will be required to reveal genetic test results to insurers or employers (Wallace 2005b). In addition, studies of the genetics of diet-related disease and appetite can detract from the social and economic factors that lead to poor health in marginalised populations (Montana 2007; Paradies et al 2007). Unless genetic testing is genuinely useful to guide treatment, promoting genetic explanations for diet-related disease can be counter-productive – wrongly implying that nothing can be done to change the situation.

Discussion

The vision of personalised diets implies that everyone should eat a different diet, based on their genes (and perhaps on other tests of their metabolism). Further, it implies that people should trust genetic testing companies and food manufacturers to tell them what their ideal diet is – implying that people should simply follow the expert recommendations and consume the products sold to them on the basis of their test results (Chadwick 2004; Meijboom et al 2003). Much of the language used to promote genetic testing in the United States claims people have a right to know their genetic risk status as a precondition of informed choice. Understanding gene-environment interactions is seen to enhance risk assessment and provide an informed basis for exposure con-

trol and lifestyle adjustments for those deemed to be at risk. But this genetic world-view promotes genetic categories as more important than
other social categories and masks the role of different powerful interests (Petersen 2003).

The global food industry clearly has an interest in promoting the concepts of individual genetic susceptibility, personalised nutrition (or medicine), and the potential role of individual nutrients in optimising
health. Yet due to biological complexity, the evidence suggests that the
'individually tailored diet' is more of a marketing concept than a scientific one, and most personal genetic information relating to common,
complex diseases is more appropriately described as genetic misinformation than genetic information. It has little to do with informing
choice and will not make healthier foods accessible to poorer people,
who are generally at higher risk of diet-related disease.

The marketing of nutrigenetic tests – widely seen as (at best) premature by researchers in the field – is spreading rapidly to Asia.

Two important issues arise in the context of the future market for
predictive genetic testing in Asia: (1) whether personalised nutrition
and nutritional genetics and genomics are good priorities for research;
and (2) whether health claims for genetic tests and associated products
are likely to be adequately regulated. Major concerns may arise in both
these areas. Unregulated genetic testing, combined with functional
foods or dietary advice, has significant potential to undermine the
health of populations, in Asia and elsewhere, by confusing healthy eating messages. In addition, resources – including research resources –
may be diverted from more valuable approaches.

The aim of tailoring diets to an individual's genetic test results
ignores the social and economic context of food production and the politics of food. An alternative aim for nutritional science is 'to contribute
to a world in which present and future generations fulfil their human
potential, live in the best of health, and develop, sustain and enjoy an
increasingly diverse human, living and physical environment' (Beauman et al 2005). This approach recognises the importance of social and
environmental issues, such as where food comes from, and the importance of improving the health of populations, not just of individuals. In
Asia, as elsewhere, such approaches might well include recognition of
the value of regional cuisines, for both health (Wahlqvist et al 2004)
and the economy (Walsh & Li 2004).

12 The Asian Genome: Racing in an Age of Pharmacogenomics

Sandra Soo-Jin Lee

In this era after the completion of the Human Genome Project (HGP), the production of genetic information through the rise of gene mapping technologies has provoked new questions regarding current models of health, identity and choice. Much focus of such hope has been on the field of pharmacogenomics, which uses genome sequencing techniques to identify the single base pair differences called single nucleotide polymorphisms (SNPs), believed to contribute to variation in drug response among individuals. Despite the seemingly ubiquitous conclusion of the HGP that humans share over 99 per cent of their genetic material, researchers of the post-HGP era are increasingly focused on the average 0.01 per cent difference between two individuals. Driving this search for meaningful differences is the promise of individualised medicines tailored to specific genetic signatures that will presumably increase efficacy and decrease toxicity.

The collection of DNA samples from global populations is aimed at identifying pharmacogenomic markers that will directly influence the direction of pharmacogenomic research in producing commercially attractive products. Implicit in the focus on pharmacogenomics is the assumption that all will stand to benefit from such investments in genomic research. While several nations, including the US, have recently focused on persistent health disparities among racially and ethnically identified populations (Smedley et al 2002), there has been little discussion of the potential impact of genomic technologies on global health disparities. The question remains as to what impact genomics will have on growing differences in health status among populations throughout the globe. While there have been increasing efforts to conduct clinical trials in non-Western nation-states, the overwhelming majority of pharmaceutical research and development continues to occur in the United States and Europe.

This chapter explores the ethical and social implications of pharmacogenomic development and the emerging framework of genetically ascribed Asian identities, and the possibility of an increasingly racialised global context where genes determine national, racial and ethnic identity. As an anthropologist interested in the institutionalisation of difference and its implications for meanings of social and cultural identity, I explore how the infrastructure for identifying population differences in human genetic variation research emerges from deeply embedded notions of where difference is most likely to be found. I am concerned with the questions of how the availability of DNA samples from specific populations in Asia affect how we understand race as related to genetics and its impact on scientific research and discovery of population specific markers of drug response. What is the impact of capital investment by multinational pharmaceutical corporations on the types of pharmaceutical products that might be tailored to Asian societies? How will investment in pharmacogenomic development in Asia come to bear on ongoing global disparities in healthcare? In grappling with these questions, this chapter discusses current trends, impediments and possibilities in pharmacogenomics and the development of therapeutics intended to be more efficacious and less toxic in Asian individuals. Of particular concern are the institutional forces that contribute to emerging fault lines of population-based therapeutics and its impact on the ability of individuals to reap the promised benefits of genomic medicine.

This chapter emerges from fieldwork conducted among scientists working on pharmacogenomic problems and from a review of the pharmacogenomic literature. In working at the intersection of anthropology and bioethics, this chapter focuses on the ethical implications of the impact of genomic sequencing technologies on concepts of group and national identity, and the interpretation of population differences in human genetic variation research.[1]

Why pharmacogenomics? The genomic promise and personalised medicine

The field of pharmacogenomics builds on genomic technologies and human genetic variation research, in creating 'tailored therapeutics' that minimise adverse drug reactions (ADRs) and maximise drug efficacy. It is well recognised that most drug therapies exhibit wide variability among individuals in their efficacy and toxicity. A study conducted in the US estimated that over 100,000 patients die and 2.2 million are injured annually by ADRs. The incidence of serious and fatal cases in hospitalised patients is reported at 6-7 per cent, making ADRs the fourth leading cause of death in the US (Lazarou et al 1998).

Currently, most new drugs are approved after clinical trials averaging only 1,500 patient exposures, usually for relatively short periods of time. Several drugs cause serious ADRs at very low frequencies that would require many more exposures to detect. To reliably discover the toxic effects of a drug with a 1 in 20,000 frequency of producing an ADR, a clinical trial would need to include at least 100,000 patient exposures. Currently, negative effects from such medications are monitored only after prescribed to patients. On a case-by-case basis, clinicians will adjust dosage and treatment type according to the reported reactions in individual patients. This 'trial and error' approach has been criticised for exposing patients to potentially harmful drug therapies, as well as exacting inefficient use of costly clinical consultation time. ADRs have come under greater scrutiny as an area ripe for intervention with the use of genetic sequencing technologies through pharmacogenomic screening. The promise of pharmacogenomics is allowing individuals to receive the 'right' medication as dictated by their unique genetic signatures, thus minimizing the need to try several medications and/or doses to achieve the desired effect.

The pharmaceutical industry, which invests approximately US $ 24 billion in research and development of new drug therapies annually, views pharmacogenomics with great interest because of its potential to produce more efficient and effective medications. The estimated savings could be upwards of 60 per cent of current costs, which now average US $ 880 million to bring a drug from bench to market (Mehl & Santell 2000). The savings are not limited to the pharmaceutical industry, but are expected to dramatically decrease the overall cost of healthcare in the US, where approximately US $ 76.6 billion is spent on drug-related morbidity and mortality (Johnson & Bootman 1995). By identifying narrow populations that may benefit from these individual drugs, pharmaceutical companies may be able to salvage these drugs by identifying and marketing them directly to a market niche of those who may presumably benefit most. While still in its nascent stages, increasing interest within academia and the pharmaceutical industry has resulted in significant investment in pharmacogenomic research.

At the heart of these efforts is a focus on human genetic variation and the identification of subpopulations which experience differing reactions to pharmaceutical products. In a time when gene therapy research has been stifled by setbacks, pharmacogenomics has become a focal point, as the first tangible deliverable on the multimillion investment of the HGP. In the absence of cost-effective whole genome sequencing capability, pharmacogenomic researchers leverage what they know about population differences and patterns of SNPs distinguishing continental groups from each another to determine the best gene candidates for drug responses of interest. The result of such a focus is reflected in a growing literature on genetic differences among groups identified as Caucasians, Africans and East Asians, each reflecting significantly different drug responses. Analysis of frequency differences of alleles associated with the metabolism of drug agents indicate that, while certain therapeutics will be efficacious in one group, they may prove ineffective or toxic in others.

The reality of the predicted era of pharmacogenomics could unfold along a number of trajectories, which are largely dependent on the institutional and industrial infrastructure being built around basic research, clinical trial studies and potential consumer markets. As opposed to the blockbuster model of 'one size fits all', pharmacogenomic development is predicated on axes of distinction that reconcile the search for salient genetic variants for drug development with potential capital gain. While the rhetoric around pharmacogenomics has been focused on individuals, a more realistic view is that 'populations' will be the unit of analysis of interest in the foreseeable future (Daar & Singer 2005). While some have argued that patterns of genetic variants irrespective of racial identification should be the driver in identifying pertinent patient populations, race has become a particularly attractive differentiating tool. As one research scientist remarked during an interview at the annual meeting on pharmacogenomics sponsored by the US-based Cold Spring Harbor Labs and Wellcome Trust in the UK:

> To say that pharmacogenomics is going to bring us an era of personalised medicine is perhaps a false statement ... more likely is population-based medicine where our knowledge of racial differences will be quite useful. It [race] may be a proxy but it remains the best interim method of stratifying populations.

If race is to be used as proxy for biomarkers, it begs the question of how individuals are to be identified with racial groups. Without explicit guidance, researchers are left to determine these answers on their own. An example is found in research on the cytochrome P450 enzymes, known to have significant influence on a broad spectrum of drugs. Several studies have cited that the cytochrome P450 variants, such as the CYP2C family of enzymes known to be active in the metabolism of warfarin, a commonly prescribed anticoagulant medication, differ significantly in frequency among populations identified as black, Caucasian and Asian. How individuals are identified within these broad categories is a question raised by many scholars. Researchers differ widely in categorization practices; some allow self-identification by participants, others ask for the continental origins of grandparents, and still others rely on researcher observation and discretion.

Lack of clear guidance is put into stark relief by the recent decision by the US Food and Drug Administration (FDA) to approve the antihypertensive medication, BiDil, for use exclusively in 'self-identified African-American patients'. This unusual decision provides evidence of the incorporation of race as a stratifying technique, where genetic variation

is often conflated as simply 'racial' and health providers are left to interpret the label on their own. By circumscribing the drug for exclusive
use by a uniquely American category of African-Americans, the debate
over the relationship between race and the body is reignited, begging
the question of what the downstream implications may be for a world
market overwhelmingly dominated by American research built on local
and historically embedded notions of racial difference. What are the
long-term effects of DNA repositories that use racial taxonomies in the
sorting of DNA, and of networks of regulatory bodies that support and
even require racial difference to be explicitly reported in all government-funded research? How does the institutionalisation of race affect
the development of the field of pharmacogenomics for other nation-
states?

Configuring global diversity and the category of 'Asian'

The pendulum shift from a dominant ethos that humans are overwhelmingly genetically similar to one that emphasises differences is reflected in how genome sequencing projects choose their research populations. In October 2002, the National Human Genome Research Institute (NHGRI) ended speculation on what would follow the HGP by
announcing the launch of the International HapMap Project. In its
press release, the institute recapitulated that the genetic sequence of
any two individuals is 99.9 per cent identical, but follows this with the
statement that 'variations may greatly affect an individual's disease risk'.
The institute describes the strategy of haplotype mapping as an efficient
approach to identifying SNPs associated with complex diseases and
drug response. Haplotype mapping is based on the idea that sets of
nearby SNPs on the same chromosome are inherited in blocks. The various patterns of SNPs on a block are haplotypes. Although these may
contain a large number of SNPs, only a few SNPs, referred to 'tag
SNPs', are enough to uniquely identify the haplotypes in a particular
block. Reducing the number of SNPs that must be identified to a smaller number of tag SNPs reduces the amount of genome to be examined
to locate the area of interest. In creating a haplotype map, the institute
is attempting to capture common haplotypes that may be used in genetic association studies of disease and drug response. The International
HapMap was expected to be an important resource in the development
of pharmacogenomics.

    The International HapMap, unlike the HGP, includes several popula-
tions identified by racial and ethnic categories. Explaining its rationale
for studying multiple populations, the institute issued the following

statement, highlighting the dual concerns over representation and justice:

> Including only one, non-disadvantaged, population would also
> avoid some of the ethical issues raised by identifying popula-
> tions. However, this approach would raise serious issues of jus-
> tice, since only that population could receive the population-
> specific advantages of the haplotype map ... The haplotype map
> should be developed so that it would be useful for mapping
> genes in any population. (NHGRI 2001)

By employing this strategy, the institute attempted to balance the demand by researchers for a timely reference map that captures genetic
diversity with the need to address ethical issues around obtaining samples from racially and/or ethnically identified populations. From the
outset of the International HapMap Project, several leading scientists
had suggested that the reference map could be created using an already
existing collection of DNA taken from individuals identified as northern
European residing in the state of Utah. This collection is referred to as
the CEPH samples. Using these samples would have eliminated the
need to conduct additional sampling and the time and energy required
to obtain proper informed consent. As one molecular biologist com-
mented, during an interview conducted for this research, 'Using the
CEPH data would save us from having to jump through the hoops of
procuring samples from sensitive places.'

The institute's statement above alludes to this in discounting the use
of 'only one, non-disadvantaged, population'. During an interview, an
International HapMap working group member stated this more directly,
suggesting that 'it would never go over politically in this day and age to
create a publicly funded map using only white people.' In the end, the
institute decided on four principle populations for inclusion in the
map: individuals from China and Japan, the Yoruba in Nigeria and the
existing collection of CEPH samples from individuals with origins in
northern Europe (www.genome.gov/10005340). What is puzzling from
the standpoint of the existing scientific literature on global patterns of
human genetic variation at the time is that individuals from China and
Japan appear to exhibit similar patterns of allelic frequencies, which are
difficult to distinguish in blind DNA sequencing studies (Rosenberg et
al 2002). Given that only four populations were included in the International HapMap, the decision to sample individuals from both China
and Japan as opposed to choosing additional African populations, which
are believed to exhibit the most genetic variation, seems to undermine
the dual goals of representation and justice outlined explicitly by the institute.

However, decisions regarding population sampling are not wholly dependent on the logic of research protocols but are borne out of sociopolitical and economic concerns. When asked about the sampling strategy of the HapMap, Francis Collins, the head of the NHGRI, stated candidly that both 'China and Japan were willing to provide monetary support for their participation in the project'.[2] The process by which nation-states are invited to participate in large, publicly funded DNA repositories reflect a larger political economy that plays directly on issues of global participation and representation in the emerging genomic age. While the support of the Chinese and Japanese governments may have produced a more 'inclusive' resource, the 'pay your way' sampling strategy may have deep repercussions on the future trajectories of research on human genetic variation, disease and drug response. While admittedly not an exhaustive reflection of global diversity, the HapMap is expected to be a pivotal resource for scientists who are interested in identifying potentially significant variations in genetic patterns. A major challenge for pharmacogenomic research and genetic association studies, in general, is the ability to produce enough 'power' to discern meaningful differences between populations. The International HapMap is emblematic of the major repositories in the public domain that reflect a skewed pattern of diversity. For example, these collections hold samples predominantly from individuals of Han Chinese and Japanese ancestry that are often lumped into the broad category of 'Asian', despite the limited representation of populations on the Asian continent.

Understanding what the category of Asian means in human genetic variation is instructive of how population differences are highly circumscribed by material challenges of obtaining samples and characterising them for the purposes of research. In their review of the literature on classes of CYP2C variants, Xie et al (2001) reported significant differences in distribution among populations. Pooling data from pharmacogenetic research in their meta-analysis, Xie et al deconstruct the broad category of 'Asian' into the three subpopulations reflected by the majority of studies. Despite the larger set of populations the category of Asian would connote, the researchers found that the three predominant study populations were Chinese, Japanese and Korean, with little representation from South and South-east Asia

The long-term effects of this sampling trend on emerging research on drug response may produce knowledge that ignores salient genetic variants among populations elsewhere in Asia, away from the centres of capital and political power. The reality is that the samples identified as 'Asian' circulating in the drug development arena have narrow origins and reflect the socio-political constraints on the global supply of DNA samples. This may have a profound effect on decisions of which drugs become tailored for which populations, as well as the production of knowledge on what is meaningful genetic difference. Perhaps most worrisome is that ongoing health disparities among populations within Asia may be deemed of tertiary importance.

National genomes and destabilising the category of 'Asian'

The global distribution of efforts towards drug development, combined with the increasingly narrow representation of DNA samples incorporated into significant genetic repositories, such as the International HapMap, sets us on a defined trajectory of pharmacogenomics. A fundamental question that is being addressed, albeit in an inexplicit way, is how difference created outside of the US/European landscape influences the development of pharmacogenomics. Another question is: how does the category of Asian influence the types of pharmacogenomic research being conducted?

It is, perhaps, not surprising that the predominant axes of differentiation fall along national lines. The creation of tailored drugs dovetails with beliefs of population-based genetic specificity particularly resonant in East Asian countries. In South Korea, the biotechnology company Macrogen announced its efforts to map the 'Korean genome', on an assumption that it is qualitatively different from the human genomes already sequenced through collaborative efforts in the US. In reporting on the Korean genome project in the Korean daily newspaper *Chosun Ilbo*, Macrogen is reported as justifying the project by stating that the 'the successful drafting of the (Korean) map follows the announcement of the successful mapping of genomes for *Caucasians* done by Celera Genomics,' Celera being a US bioengineering company, in June of last year [emphasis added] (Cha 2004). Contrary to assertions that the HGP was a map applicable to all humans, the Korean genome effort reflects an understanding of the HGP applicable only to whites. This reading of the HGP map reflects the chasms that divide genomic science despite its context of increasing globalisation. The lingering east-west racial divide is clear in the *raison d'être* for the Korean genome, and forges notions of significant genetic differences among racially identified populations; but it also asserts that realisation of the pharmacogenomic dream must occur locally. Implicit in its rationale of the project are notions of purity and particularity. On Macrogen's website, the company states:

> As Korea has a strong tendency to propagate within its race, Korea maintains relatively pure blood pool as compared with members of other nations. So, we expect that a study of several participants' genome structure will give us a Korean-specific genome structure. This project will also help us to obtain Korean

genomic blue prints including patterns of single nucleotide polymorphisms (SNPs). The results of the Korean genome project
will be the basis for developing personalized medicine in the
near future. (www.macrogen.com/english/index.html [accessed
11.10.03])

The rationale for a separate Korean genome project rests on the assumption that without a 'Korean genomic blueprint', the anticipated
benefits of the new genetics will not materialise. The argument that a
national DNA project is essential in order to create 'personalised medicines' reflects the reinscription of individual genomes into a national,
yet personalised, racial category that is framed as distinct from other
'racial types' already sequenced. The goal, according to company president Suh Jeong-Seon, is to 'decode the biological definition of the word
'Korean" (http://kn.koreaherald.co.kr/SITE/data/html_dir/2001/06/30/
200106300007.asp [accessed 11.10.03]), making the claim that the elu-
sive essence of Korean identity resides in genes, and sequencing is critical to understanding and treating the Korean body. It is in this construction of genes that processes of racialisation occur where difference is
understood as both inherent and prescriptive.

Sequencing projects that attempt to create a nationalised genome
crystallise what constitutes the national body and whom that includes.
In the autumn of 2007, scientists from the Beijing Genome Institute
reported that they had completed a full sequence of an individual identified as Han Chinese (Borell 2007). Announcements focused upon the
potential pharmacogenomic benefits:

> Although humans share most of their genome with one another,
> slight genetic differences may correspond to variation in their
> susceptibility to diseases and responses to therapeutics. Han Chi-
> nese represent 92 per cent of China's population and are the lar-
> gest ethnic group in the world. People in the same ethnic groups
> can share genetic characteristics that may be useful for targeting
> future drug treatments.

This project continues in an effort by the BGI to sequence the entire
genomes of 100 individuals over three years. Named the Yunhuang Project, in honour of two emperors thought to be the ancestors of the Han
Chinese, China's largest ethnic group, the national project reinscribes
Han lineage as national identity. Addressing concerns over capturing
the genomes of other ethnic groups, Ye Jia, a spokeswoman for the project, said that once the project is completed, the BGI aims to sequence
the genomes of thousands more people, including ethnic groups from
other Asian countries. For now, the Yunhuang Project, like the Interna-

tional HapMap Project, focuses on the Han Chinese. Heralded as one of the first international projects to focus on the whole genomes of private individuals, it has been reported that one individual paid as much as 10 million yuan (approximately US $ 1.4 million) to have his genome sequenced (Qiu & Hayden 2008). The role of individual capital in driving the genomic revolution towards personalised medicine deserves greater attention, in the context of the promise for broad participation and universal benefit in the near future.

Clinical trials: the impact of bridge studies

The rise of national genome projects focusing on 'population differences' emerges as part of a larger continuum of practices in drug development that suggest not all groups can be treated the same. The focus on national and, indeed, racial specificity is perhaps no better institutionalised in the context of drug development than in Japan. Japan remains a frontrunner in asserting racial difference in drug response and requires 'bridge studies' to be conducted on approved drugs tested on other populations by pharmaceutical companies in the US and Europe. The Japanese Ministry of Health and Welfare has argued for the necessity of bridge studies, to demonstrate both efficacy and safety of drugs for the Japanese population, making the claim that without local data, no reasonable assurances could be made about biological differences between the Japanese and the rest of the world. Recently, the Japanese government mandated a pharmacogenomic analysis of all drugs currently on the market and being used in the Japanese population to determine the genetic underpinnings for why their population may react differently to drugs that have been clinically tested on populations in the United States and Europe.

Undergirding these regulatory controls is a prima facie belief in inherent biological and genetic differences that resonate with claims made in South Korea and China regarding national genome sequencing efforts. Such ideology on difference, combining biological with cultural understandings of national identity, can have a serious impact on the infrastructure within which pharmacogenomics is conducted. Japan has the second largest pharmaceutical market in the world, with US $ 46.82 billion in sales, or 19 per cent of the global market. The pharmaceutical market in Japan is larger than in any other country except for the US, where sales amount to US $ 87.72 billion, or 35 per cent of the global market. This is daunting when one considers that most of this economic activity is directed toward the domestic market of Japanese nationals. Even as a reification of national boundaries occurs within the context of global development of pharmacogenomic products, so too do the emerging national fault lines reproduce the illusion of genetic homogeneity within national borders.

What is at stake?

Lisa Gannet describes a shift in language in the 1950s that signalled a retreat away from the scientific racism which defined earlier eugenic research. Anthropologists and other social scientists promulgated new models of race as socially constructed and defined by historical and political context. The field of genetics, suffering from a previous era of using science conducted in highly regarded scientific institutions, including the Cold Spring Harbor Laboratories in the US, to justify the exploitation and condemnation of groups, followed the lead of Theodosius Dobzhansky in replacing 'race' with 'population'. However, the shift to 'populational thinking' according to Gannett (2001) retains a framework of hierarchical difference in a calculus of human qualities mapped onto discrete classifications. The efforts in South Korea, China and Japan to differentiate the genome along national lines, in order to discover genetic variants that are functionally useful, reflect a durable research infrastructure built upon the notion of racial difference. As the natural offspring of a political economy of drug development which retains specific centres of power and activity, national projects in Japan, South Korea and China articulate a rhetorical logic linking national identity, race and biological specificity.

However, questions remain as to the utility of such investments. In the search for common variants causing common diseases such as coronary heart disease, diabetes, depression and other conditions, are such projects that attempt to glean national and putatively distinct DNA the best use of efforts within the global context? Will the discovery of different genetic associations for drugs used to alleviate common diseases challenge our current notion of *human* diseases that affect all populations? Will such notions of particularity challenge definitions of common diseases and result in the emergence of distinct forms of medication, e.g. different pills/dosages for medication to treat Korean depression as opposed to Japanese? How does an infrastructure of research that presupposes group difference put into motion trajectories of inquiry that recapitulate ideas of distinct groups divided along not genetic, but political and social, lines?

The anticipated utopia of pharmacogenomics is founded upon the expectation that access to genetically tailored drugs will be available to the general public and will address genetic variation among subpopulations. However, the infrastructure for the pharmacogenomic revolution as it is currently being constructed reflects an accentuation of the global polarity that exists in the production, distribution and compensation of drugs. With 90 per cent of drug development sponsored by the United States, Europe and Japan, few other countries participate in this dialogue.

In lieu of using national categories or continental categories, individuals will need to be tested for pharmacogenomic specificity. The development of such tools is largely impeded by a population-based lens guided by the political economy of global drug development. The current trajectory is the development of local drugs for local populations that dovetails with the ways in which pharmacogenomic data are currently collected. Defining patient populations along national, racial and ethnic lincs, not surprisingly, conflates genetics with national, racial and ethnic phenomena. The current infrastructure of research does not assure that drugs which work better on Koreans will be as effective for a subset of individuals in Indonesia and Botswana. Given the current dominant prism of difference through which variants are identified, this question is left unanswered and these drugs may never be offered to those individuals.

The racialisation of pharmacogenomic development through sampling strategies and ideologies of difference, institutionalised both in and outside Asia, has produced national fault lines that circumvent human genetic variation research possibly revealing the highly integrated patterns exhibited in global populations. The stakes in this occlusion are not merely academic. Despite the much-heralded promise of individualised medicine, the current trajectory of the genomic revolution may prevent any serious engagement with ongoing global disparities in disease burden and suffering. While there are many concerns over genetic sampling of populations, the current practice of extrapolating from narrow sets of East Asian samples under the broader category of Asian leaves little hope that researchers will discover pharmacogenomic products that may be more efficacious and less toxic for many populations in Asia. The answer to the question of who will reap the benefits of genomically tailored medicine begs a further fundamental question of whether, in a time when basic improvements in hygiene and public health infrastructure are needed for so many individuals, worldwide genomic screening of populations for pharmacogenomic drug products is a just and defensible investment.

Notes

1 This research was funded by a Mentored Scientist Development Award in Research Ethics from the National Human Genome Research Institute #K01 HL72465.
2 Personal communication, meeting of the International Society for Pharmacogenomics, Los Angeles.

13 Discussion: Predictive and Genetic Testing in Asian and International Contexts

Margaret Sleeboom-Faulkner

Introduction

This concluding chapter provides a comparative overview of themes crucial to the frameworks in which choices regarding predictive genetic testing (PGT) are made, and central to the chapters in this volume. At the same time, it views the particular practices associated with these themes, e.g. the marketing of tests by commercial companies, and testing interventions, in a critical light. The themes central to the frameworks of choice regarding predictive and genetic testing in Asia are: 'free' will; the therapeutic gap; the role of the state; culture and discrimination; the role of the market; and global developments and PGT. The concept of the framework of choice here is meant to shed light on and emphasise the role of contexts and situations in which choices are made, experienced and considered as free, individual, communal or conditional.

Reproductive governance is shaped in and by the minds of social individuals and the regulatory decisions of the state. Foucault indicated that individuals and society in this context are two sides of the same productive process, shaped interactively and simultaneously, so that their development cannot be understood independent of the other (Novas & Rose 2000). For this reason, the notion of the 'free will' of individuals can only be understood in the context in which it is used. Nevertheless, the ways in which individuals and states relate to one another differs per society. Consequently, the notion of 'free will' in reproductive choice and choices regarding PGTs may also be experienced differently in nation-states with different relations between the individual and the state. For instance, in some social contexts, people tend to favour the idea of having a free will, even though this 'free' will is shaped and constrained by numerous factors. Given that the individual at the same time is constituted by state and community norms, governance of genetic and predictive testing and screening takes place within the particular constraints of varying cultural, financial, social, state and international environments.

For individuals in different societies, then, a variety of possibilities and histories yields various prospects and opportunities, which individuals and groups may be aware of, depending on factors such as individual ability, social connections, education, and the availability of information through commercial and state media. The question of whether and how they use opportunities has much to do with the way in which they weigh their advantages (preference), existing norms (cultural customs and official regulation) and perceptions of risk (Beck 1992; 2007; Adam 2007). The interaction of these frameworks of choice and the various constellations of perceived, presented and taken opportunities and risks form a dynamic and ever-changing range of factors defining situations in which major reproductive choices are made and their consequences unfold. These frameworks and ramifications of choice regarding genetic and predictive testing are the main themes of this book, explored in two large developing countries – China and India; a small developing country – Sri Lanka; and a wealthy welfare society – Japan. Comparing the frameworks/ramifications of choice in these societies, it has become clear that the relevant problematic in these four countries differs along distinct fault lines: wealth, healthcare provision, the role of the state, and indigenous cultures and religions. Below is a discussion of the six recurring themes in this volume, which form the parameters of the frameworks and ramifications of choice: 'free' will; the therapeutic gap; the role of the state; culture and discrimination; the role of the market; and global developments and PGT.

Constituent factors of frameworks of choice

Free will/choice in the termination of pregnancy

The theme of free will/choice is expressed in debates regarding PGT and abortion after prenatal testing, involving issues of the 'slippery slope' argument, the question of when one should speak of coercion, pressure, or free will, the interdependency of people, and the issue of choice avoidance. The 'slippery slope' argument claims that by transgressing a boundary norm or threshold – setting aside one principle – a process is set in motion that is hard to stop, leading to undesirable results. In the context of 'designer babies' (Silver 1999; Stock 2002), the application of this principle would mean that the selection of a foetus or embryo, on the basis of a certain trait, would lead to a society in which people are no longer valued in and of themselves (Kant 1996; Döring). Against this slippery slope claim it is argued that people, if they want to, can always halt such a process and exercise their free choice to stop undesirable effects of the process concerned (Harris 1997; Savulescu 1999b). It seems likely that both sides of the argument have a point, depending on the circumstances of application and the nature of the societal forces at work. In a situation where state policy, available technology and community conspire to put pressure onto couples in one direction, one could indeed imagine a slippery slope at work – the question is to what extent individuals and society as a whole are able to steer and halt processes of change in this field. It is also quite usual, however, that in a given society a constellation of pressures go in different directions, leaving space for couples and individuals to mould their decisions and back-up plans accordingly.

However, the question of whether one should speak of coercion or free will, and how various pressures are experienced and interpreted, remains unsolved. There is a range of pressures that one could place on a continuum from coercion to free will. Thus, the participation in sickle cell anaemia (SCA) screening in some Indian communities is decided by the community leaders and is experienced as coercive (Patra & Sleeboom-Faulkner). Alternatively, the religious background to the regulation of reproductive decisions on pregnancy termination in some Buddhist and Christian circles might sanction boundary transgression through ostracisization, mental pressure, and penal measures (Simpson). Furthermore, the close-knit and interdependent nature of family households in some countries makes it nearly impossible for an individual to make reproductive decisions without being conscious of the wishes of family members and the consequences of going against the grain of community values (Gupta).

It is not always clear if the experience of free will should be interpreted as such. For, in a modern welfare society, where women may like to think that they can make decisions independently, one still has to view their decisions within a social context. For instance, in Japan some women think they make up their own mind about undergoing a test for ultrasound and amniocentesis through information from magazines, family and so on, not realising that information is often skewed and provided in the context of certain birthing norms and policies. Some tests have unexpectedly far-reaching consequences. So-called fun-scans, taken out of curiosity or to raise the husband's awareness of his (potential) parenthood, might force couples into a position to abort when fetal abnormality is revealed unexpectedly (Tsuge). In other situations, again, people try to avoid decision-making with respect to reproduction or taking tests, sometimes to hold on to notions of healthy 'family stock' or descent (Kato). The conscious choice 'not to know' is one that becomes increasingly difficult in societies that value healthy offspring of a certain kind or gender, although the contest between forces against selective abortion, such as the disability movement in Japan and anti-sex selection policies in China, make for a continuously shifting fault line of acceptability (Rose 2003) in all the countries examined in this volume.

Therapeutic gaps

The concept of the therapeutic gap was central to many of the accounts in this volume, and refers to the space that opens up as a result of the lacunae between the availability of predictive tests and knowledge and the possible means of dealing with the predicted condition (Holtzman & Shapiro 1998). These lacunae appear in different forms, varying from religious and cultural to economic and regulatory spaces. Thus, when testing facilities are available for prenatal testing or genetic screening, but people positively diagnosed are not in a position to have an abortion, or if no medicine or therapy is available, then we speak of a therapeutic gap. For instance, when diagnosed with thalassaemia, the high cost of chelation therapy and blood transfusion for the poor in India and China opens up one kind of therapeutic gap (Gupta). For the same reason, participation in SCA screening in some Indian communities leaves a treatment gap (Patra & Sleeboom-Faulkner). A therapeutic gap is also opened up, however, if religious values or regulation in the name of religion prevent those tested from taking remedial measures, such as the termination of pregnancy (Simpson).

Many testing facilities, being expensive, are not available in developing countries or are accessible to a small minority of the population. Thus, predictive testing for various hereditary cancer syndromes is (sorely) lacking in India, Sri Lanka and China. However, in large developing countries, such as China and India, some pharmaceutical and testing companies might seek market opportunities by offering genetic tests, dietary medicine, and therapies in the hope of attracting the patronage of a growing middle class. With a lack of health services and insurance coverage, this also opens up therapeutic gaps among even the relatively wealthy. In China, to families with a child suffering from Duchenne muscular dystrophy (DMD), this can lead to desperate actions, such as begging doctors to include them in clinical trials for new drugs or seeking alternatives in traditional Chinese medicine (TCM) (Sui & Sleeboom-Faulkner). In other cases, patients and their families seek consolation or help in religion or astrology (Simpson, Saxena and others).

The role of the state

The role of the state in practices regarding PGTs may take on different forms, varying from its regulatory function in formulating and supervising the practices of PGTs, its political role in health provision, its role as a distributor of financial resources, and its role in the minds of people. The way the state regulates PGT is important to the way testing is conducted, how testing results are dealt with, and how genetic counselling takes place. For example, the formulation of policies in the People's Republic of China (PRC) to prevent new cases of DMD in practice augments the discrimination of families with DMD. The stigma attached to DMD is the result of a policy that encourages carrier testing for DMD, on the one hand, and a policy that tries to rid society of the birth of children with DMD, on the other. Such policies discourage carrier testing among risk groups looking to avoid stigmatisation. State policies in the PRC in the case of prenatal testing, however, insist on the autonomy of the patient to make decisions about abortion. Despite the clear regulatory avoidance of compulsion, patients are expected to follow the advice of the 'genetic counsellor' (Döring, Sui & Sleeboom-Faulkner).

Apart from directly regulating PGTs, the state's role as a population policymaker and healthcare provider has a great impact on PGTs in practice. In the PRC, the population and family planning policies have led couples to desire their child to be of 'high quality', and in many areas a preference for boys has led to a gender gap (Döring, Gupta). In Sri Lanka, however, the strict religious policies on abortion mean that couples use prenatal testing not so much to terminate a pregnancy but to prepare for the birth of a disabled infant (Simpson). Though in some cases there are clear discrepancies between state policies and popular views on abortion and predictive testing, sometimes it is hard to draw a clear dividing line between the two. In both the PRC and India, there are strict guidelines against gender selection, putting both mothers and physicians under pressure not to abort potential daughters. In practice, however, public views in local communities, especially among some castes and cultural groups in India, and in rural areas in China, privilege families with sons (Gupta, Döring). Although women and physicians are held responsible for gender selection, the whole family and community can be involved in the decision-making. State policies and public views sometimes reinforce each other unintentionally. Thus, the recognition in China of the importance of having a male in rural households, by allowing a second child if the first is a girl, has made the policies against sex selection and the discrimination of women hard to swallow in rural areas, actually aggravating it. In short, although there may be very clear boundaries between state policies, public opinion, and private aims, it is not always possible to delineate them from one another in practice and to trace their combined effects.

To complicate matters further, the role the state plays in people's minds may vary with the actual role played by the state in practice. Thus, in China, healthcare provision is advertised as 'serving the people', even though the healthcare system has collapsed since the 1980s, and even though progressively less funding has been funnelled into the healthcare system (Yang 2008). This 'socialist' image is still quoted as a reason for underpaying medical doctors, which has led to widespread corruption in this sector otherwise run on the basis of market principles. Especially considering that doctors can receive bonuses for using certain high-tech procedures, the use of genetic tests classified as high-tech in some cases has been the subject of criticism. In the case of Japan, similarly, the role of the state has been and is still perceived to be a source of eugenic policies, and has driven women's groups to collaborate with handicapped groups out of solidarity against the systematic annihilation of handicapped foetuses (Tsuge, Kato). To what extent current state policies warrant such solidarity, however, is disputable.

Cultures of discrimination?

It is clear that in the societies studied in this volume, stigma and the fear of discrimination play an important role in the decision to undergo PGT. The decision to take a carrier test, prenatal test, screening or a symptomatic test is largely made on the basis of fears of becoming an object of discrimination, be it oneself, one's child, one's family or even one's tribe or community. Thus, premarital testing in China is problematic to individuals who are in doubt about their health situation, fearing that carriership of, for instance, hepatitis is revealed (Wu 2007). Prenatal testing may be done to avoid carrying the stigma of having a handicapped child in Japan, and also a daughter in China and India, while in Sri Lanka a prenatal test among religiously inclined groups evidently would serve the preparation of the family for life with a handicapped child. In Sri Lanka and Japan, however, not taking a test apparently may be motivated by 'life affirming' reasons, linked to religion or humanist attitudes. In some Chinese environments, it was found that the idea that a family member has a handicap might lead to stigmatisation of the entire household, with consequences for marriage possibilities, social status, and daily livelihood. Carrier testing then is a very sensitive business, as there is much at stake for both the person entering the family (usually the woman) and the household itself (Sui & Sleeboom-Faulkner). Another way in which discrimination is expressed was described in the context of both Chinese and Japanese families (Kato), where the idea that there may be a heritable syndrome in the family in some cases is so much suppressed and feared that it leads to the adoption of a strategy of test avoidance. In India, screening of tribal communities for SCA has lead to the stigmatisation of entire tribes as 'incestuous', as test results in some communities were distributed on coloured cards, symbolising the carrier status of individuals and leading to problems of stigma and hardship (Patra & Sleeboom-Faulkner).

In all four societies studied, as to whether tests were undertaken to avoid or to affirm life with a handicap, the theme of discrimination plays a central role. Kato's work also reveals that when people are highly educated in a high-tech society, such as Japan, some deliberately remain 'ignorant' of prenatal testing as a strategy for maintaining their social identity as a non-disabled person. Here, tradition is unexpectedly central to people's explanations of disability, in which 'blood', fate, and 'heaven' play a key role. In Japan, contradictory factors have made genetics a sensitive topic. Thus, creating a 'genetic underclass' through genetic testing is feared as potentially leading to unacceptable 'genetic discrimination' (Porter). Despite the widespread discrimination against the handicapped and termination of pregnancy in Japan, there is also a culture of awareness of patient rights and eugenic laws, limiting the practice of eugenic abortion. Although technological know-how is widely available, both women and gynaecologists tend to avoid disclosure of prenatal testing procedures so as to deflect criticism and discrimination of disabled people (Tsuge). Of course, one must ask the question of whether this loyalty towards the handicapped can be maintained, thanks to the availability of facilities for the handicapped and the wealth in Japanese society. Nevertheless, in comparison with the US, such loyalty plays a large role, just as solidarity with the unborn handicapped is widely voiced in Sri Lanka in a strict religious and regulatory environment.

However, especially in cultures where the continuation of the patrilineal household is emphasised and highly valued, the production of healthy male offspring tends to be an issue of pride entangled with cultural and religious customs of labour division. Although female newborns are not necessarily unwelcome in the family, household resources tend to be invested in males. In the PRC, the one-child policy for this reason has encouraged the abortion of females and abnormal foetuses alike, a trend salient in India too. Pride in the strength of the household, then, is often associated with the discrimination of females and the handicapped, a concept that may vary in meaning per country and per region. The birth of a handicapped child in tightly organised family households and communities in both China and India tends to be accompanied by stigma, discrimination, isolation, marriage problems, abandonment and the blaming of women for producing unsuitable offspring (Gupta, Patra & Sleeboom-Faulkner, Döring, Sui & Sleeboom-Faulkner).

Roles of the market

Commercial genetic testing is a controversial matter, especially in developing countries and countries without effective regulation on the practices of genetic testing. In Japan, commercial genetic testing plays a marginal role in the lives of patients, though hospitals are under obligation to adopt testing equipment when proven necessary to the patient's health and well-being and when affordable. In healthcare provision, however, it hardly plays a role, as the availability and expense of tests, drugs and therapies are carefully regulated: the state and insurance companies compensate for approved drugs and therapies. As people are generally insured, there is little room for commercial trade in genetic tests to potential patients. In a developing country such as China, regulation for prenatal testing and monogenetic diseases may be in place – commercial companies are not supposed to offer reproductive tests – but there are ample market opportunities for companies to sell their diagnostic genetic and predictive tests to customers. In particular, tests for multifactorial genetic diseases, such as forms of cancer and Alzheimer's disease, are on offer. As the development of such multifactorial genetic diseases depends on both genetic and environmental factors, predictions are hard to make. The reliability of these tests is hard to check, and the terms in which the 'test results' are reported to customers are usually vague, resembling the predictions of fortune tellers (Sui & Sleeboom-Faulkner 2007). The companies play on the hopes of people and on their belief in science, while the customers receive either an undesired result to worry about or the false certainty of a desired result. The commercial advertisements of such tests seize upon the respect many people in China have for scientific achievements, science and technology being one of the four modernisations, which the Party deems responsible for the post-1978 reforms. Foreign technology has an exceptionally 'clean' image, which is used by testing companies in Internet articles recommending the merits of their tests in quasi-scientific terms hard for non-specialists to check and verify.

In other cases, foreign pharmaceutical companies introduce advanced predictive technologies from abroad, including testing equipment and reagents. Sometimes deals are made between these companies and the government, making scientists in hospitals dependent on technologies they have to pay for dearly without being sure of their suitability to their particular situation (interview with Dr Tao (pseudonym), hospital in Shanghai, 28 April 2007). In other cases, companies are set up on the basis of collaborations between scientists with foreign networks and investors. They sell their testing kits to remote communities in the countryside for a relatively low price or even for free, enabling small clinics to diagnose hundreds of diseases in patients (interview with Dr Huang (pseudonym) in Wuhan, 20 October 2007). Receiving equipment for a low price may be advantageous for a short while, but the required reagents are expensive and, when communities have become used to the equipment and the new testing kits, there is no guarantee that prices will remain as favourable. Although the testing equipment will help some patients to find a solution to their health problems, others will not be able to afford suitable therapy, even when available. The companies themselves regard their work as a lucrative challenge to help the country advance, deriving most of their profit from deals with large city hospitals. At the same time, the kickbacks hospitals receive for making these deals partly compensate for low salaries, but also encourage the corruption-ridden state healthcare system.

In Japan, a wealthy welfare society, people receive free state healthcare. However, the percentage patients have to contribute to their healthcare bill has increased to 30 per cent, with a maximum monthly limit of around 600,000 Yen. Over half of the adult population takes extra healthcare insurance through private companies, and most family households take out a life insurance policy for the main wage-earner, usually the male head of the family. The introduction of genetic testing has made it, in principle, possible for insurance companies to pick healthy clients (cherry-picking), though they do risk clients engaging in adverse selection by choosing their life insurance on the basis of the genetic knowledge they have of themselves (Porter). Referring to several rulings by the Japanese High Court, Porter showed that insurance companies currently do not require clients to undergo genetic tests (this is still an unregulated area). Yet with hindsight, clients are responsible for their disease also if symptoms become manifest after the commencement of the contract, and even if genetic diagnosis occurs afterwards. The knotty issues of allocating 'responsibility' for diseases with a large genetic component are likely to be dealt with differently according to the rules of the healthcare model adopted in different countries. The market, no doubt, will play an important role in research, product development and marketing in all healthcare models. For, even if commercial exchanges are not directly visible to the patients, in the end, they are the ones who will shoulder the costs indirectly.

International biotechnological developments and predictive and genetic testing

One consequence of global developments is the spreading of biotechnologies and commercial products, such as testing kits and functional foods, to areas lacking basic healthcare provisions. Global commercial and scientific developments in PGTs have not just led to better predictions and an increased ability to deal with health problems; due to the unavailability of drugs, therapies, and follow-up care, combined with the discrimination and suffering of those tested positive, newly-generated medical knowledge has also become a burden. Also, in the West the question has arisen as to what extent diets and genetic testing can form a solution for people suspected to be at risk of developing multifactorial diseases, such as heart disease or Alzheimer's disease (Wallace; Lock 2005). The same question, in Asian environments, and particularly in developing countries, was shown to yield even more problems in terms of consumer safety, critical discussion on and scrutiny of health products, and the availability of healthcare (Wallace).

Pharmacogenomics aims to develop medicine for people with a certain genetic and environmental background. Though this branch of science has not met the high expectations (Martin et al 2006; Hedgecoe 2005), producers of functional foods act as if sufficient reliable knowledge were available to offer diet foods to people with a particular genetic background (Sui & Sleeboom-Faulkner 2007). Diet foods and commercial genetic tests are advertised as medical solutions for diseases in environments that are insufficiently regulated, while people are uninformed about the risks. Here, advantage is taken of what I call *technological displacement*. Scientific knowledge and technology to a certain extent evolve in a laboratory environment, and develop for application in the society for whose institutions and circumstances they have been shaped (Fujimura 1992; Hacking 1992). Transplanted into another institutional environment and circumstances, such knowledge and technology may clash with alien host institutions and harm their users. The lucrative transplantation of diet foods and testing technologies into developing societies may not be checked by traditions of critical consumer evaluation, institutionalised supervision or effective control of consumer products. Ironically, diet foods and commercial tests target relatively wealthy people, while people with actual genetic risks are not diagnosed or provided with care, as this requires more locally-situated knowledge, provisions and healthcare funding (Wallace).

One reason for conducting pharmacogenomics research is the study of the prediction of adverse drug reactions (ADRs). Knowledge of such predictions is important, because ADR is a major iatrogenic cause of death in countries that make much use of drugs in healthcare. Ideally, research on people's genetic make-up would yield information on the ADR of individuals, but high expenses associated with individual research lead geneticists to use the analytical unit of the population, or race, to determine the biomarkers for such groups of people (Sleeboom-Faulkner 2006). This scientific practice has led to various questions about the influence of such research in an international context. One of the factors generating the therapeutic gap is the investment in science and technologies with applications limited to predefined populations that are already advantaged. The use of particular research methods and agendas in particular environments then influences the ability of populations to benefit from genomic medicine.

Pharmacogenomics, although not setting out to aggravate race relations or base concepts of medicine on socio-cultural concepts of race (Wade 2002; Lee 2003), through its very activities has affected the global landscape of population divisions via the technologies and mapping exercises it employs. The HapMap project, described in Lee's chapter, for instance, is based on the genetic sampling of a limited number (five) of 'representative' regions in the world. This means that, in the long run, relevant genetic differences between otherwise defined populations will be under-researched, and that the drugs developed on the basis of certain genetic profiles may adversely affect the health of the underrepresented populations, if they reach them at all. Thus, when drugs are used in the absence of population-specific alternatives, under-researched populations may be disadvantaged, suffering adverse affects of drugs not suitable to their physical traits. This trend may also affect health disparities within Asia. Apart from consequences for healthcare provision and drugs, pharmacogenomic activities also affect issues of socio-cultural and political significance. The genetic sampling and mapping projects carried out in Asia make racial claims about the nature of various peoples in nation-states (Sung 2008; Patra & Sleeboom-Faulkner 2007; Sleeboom-Faulkner 2006). These racial claims are intimately linked to issues of health, ethnicity and national identity (Lee). As Lee indicates, racial claims are mobilised for political purposes, to create and confirm the racial and ethnic identity of nation-states. Although the delineation between the ways in which the concepts of race and ethnicity are used is often hard to make, when DNA sequencing methods and haplotyping are used to define a 'national' genome for political and economic purposes, it is clear that the concept of 'race' is given biological content. Attempts to use genomic evidence as a basis for the regulation of medical trials and drug testing in Japan can be seen as an example of the racialisation of nation-states (Kuo 2008). In such instances, the 'human genome' is used to justify racial distinction based on 'genetic averages' [sic] found in a particular nation-state. Although population-specific testing may have great safety benefits, the racial distinction made here is based on the ideological concept of the 'nation-state' as a genetically homogenous unit, and used to decide whether or not the retesting of 'foreign' drugs is necessary.

Ramifications of choice and predictive genetic tests in Asia

The frameworks in which choices are made regarding PGTs differ radically between Asian countries, the ramifications of which depend on factors related to constraints and pressures at the individual, societal and global level. At the individual level, decisions are made by individuals in relation to their families and the local community, on the basis of the freedom left to them in this context to choose to undergo PGTs, and the support they can expect for dealing with the consequences of taking tests. These decisions, in turn, depend on resources available to them, such as awareness and understanding of the use of PGTs, healthcare access and follow-up care. Apart from material and financial resources, religious and philosophical life and family values are sometimes crucial to the decision about taking a neonatal test for DMD or Down's syndrome, or to have an abortion.

This overview of studies shows that at the national level, the provision of healthcare and the financial coverage of medical therapy, the regulation of therapies, drugs and follow-up, the availability of schooling and awareness of medical possibilities, the level of scientific development and quality of hospitals, and population and family-planning policies are all part of the complex, varying frameworks which shape and are part of the decision-making process regarding the use of PGTs.

The global level of complex international networks and inequalities is difficult to delineate but is nonetheless real, and has concrete consequences for the shaping of frameworks in which societies and individuals make provisions and decisions. In the sphere of science, international scientific exchanges, collaborations and contacts, the adoption of bioethical guidelines, and the ways in which international genetic sampling projects and genomics research choose their population units were shown to frame the choices of individuals indirectly (Lee, Wallace); in the socio-economic sphere, the international availability of genetic sampling populations, the relative social and financial vulnerability of populations, and the relative bioethical permissiveness of state and local governments influence the extent to which populations participate in genetic testing and benefit from genetic sampling in a global context; in the sphere of national policymaking, the international profile of countries as accommodating of globalised research, and the manner in which nation-states shape their national bio-identity vis-à-vis other nation-states, mould the spaces and ways in which individuals make use of PGTs.

Contributors

Ole Döring
GIGA-Institute for Asian Studies, Hamburg, Germany

Jyotsna A. Gupta
University of Humanistics, Utrecht, the Netherlands

Masae Kato
Institute for Japanese Studies, Leiden University, the Netherlands

Prasanna K. Patra
International Institute of Asian Studies (IIAS), Leiden, the Netherlands

Gerard Porter
AHRC Research Centre for Studies in Intellectual Property and Technology Law, School of Law, University of Edinburgh, United Kingdom

Renu Saxena
Sir Ganga Ram Hospital, New Delhi, India

Bob Simpson
Department of Anthropology, Durham University, United Kingdom

Margaret Sleeboom-Faulkner
Department of Anthropology, Sussex University, United Kingdom

Sandra Soo-Jin Lee
Centre for Biomedical Ethics, Stanford University Medical School, United States of America

Suli Sui
Amsterdam School of Social Science Research (ASSR), University of Amsterdam, the Netherlands

Azumi Tsuge
Department of Sociology, Meijigakuin University, Tokyo, Japan

Ishwar C. Verma
Sir Ganga Ram Hospital, New Delhi, India

Helen Wallace
GeneWatch UK, United Kingdom

Bibliography

Achim, R. (2004), 'Tackling an unsolved problem: the challenge of genetic testing: new genetics and public opinion', *Journal of the Association of Life Insurance Medicine of Japan* 102 (2): 123-133.

Adam, B. (2007), 'Introduction: repositioning risk: the challenge for social theory', in B. Adam, U. Beck & J. van Loon (eds.), *The Risk Society and Beyond*, 1-31. London: Sage.

Adorno, T.W. (1951), *Minima Moralia. Reflections from a damaged life*. London: Sage.

Akerlof, G.A. (1970), 'The market for lemons: quality, uncertainty and the market mechanism', *The Quarterly Journal of Economics* 84 (3): 488-500.

Amari, K. (2006), *Iryō hoken yakkan ni okeru hōteki mondai* (Legal problems with medical insurance clauses). wwwsoc.nii.ac.jp/jsis2/documents/h18amari_r.pdf.

American Academy of Pediatrics Committee on Bioethics (AAP) (2001), 'Ethical issues with genetic testing in pediatrics', *Pediatrics* 107 (6): 1451-1455.

American College of Medical Genetics (2004), 'ACMG statement on direct-to-consumer genetic testing', *Genetics in Medicine* 6 (1): 60.

Andrews, L. (2001), *Future Perfect: Confronting decisions about genetics*. New York: Colombia University Press.

Anonymous (2001), 'China set to become world player in gene technology', *China Education and Research Network*, 1 January. www.edu.cn/20010101/22701.shtml.

Anonymous (2005), 'Dr. Ci Labo to begin home obesity gene testing service', *JCN Network*, 9 May. www.japancorp.net/Article.Asp?Art_ID=9995.

Anonymous (2006), 'Child obesity a bigger problem', *China View*, 10 July. www.chinacdc.net.cn/n272562/n276003/13244.html.

Anonymous (2008), 'New fetal DNA test stirs fresh hopes, concerns', (Washington Post), *The Japan Times*, 27 October.

Arai, M., J. Utsonomiya, & Y.Miki (2004), 'Familial breast and ovarian cancers', *International Journal of Clinical Oncology* 9: 270-282.

Arai, S. (2002), 'Global view on functional foods: Asian perspectives', *British Journal of Nutrition* 88 (Suppl. 2): S139-S143.

Arimori, N. (2005), 'Idenkango to wa? (What is genetic nursing?)'. *Josan zasshi* 59 (2): 117-122.

Armstrong, K., B. Weber, G. FitzGerald, J.C. Hershey, M.V. Pauly, J. Lemaire, K. Subramanian & D.A. Asch (2003), 'Life insurance and breast cancer risk assessment: adverse selection, genetic testing decisions, and discrimination', *American Journal of Medical Genetics* 120A: 359-364.

The Asahi Shimbun. 14 February 1996. Yûseihogohôkaisei tachiba no sa. Tokyo.

Ashcroft, R. (2007), 'Should genetic information be disclosed to insurers?', *British Medical Journal* 334: 1197.

Asian Development Bank (2007), *Moving toward knowledge-based economies*. September. www.adb.org/Documents/Reports/Technical-Notes/Knowledge-Based-Economies/knowledge-based-economies.pdf.

Baird, P. (2001), 'The Human Genome Project, genetics and health', *Community Genetics* 4: 77-80.

Baird, P. (2002), 'Identification of genetic susceptibility to common diseases: the case for regulation', *Perspectives in Biology and Medicine* 45: 516-528.

Balgir, R.S. (2001), 'Genetic epidemiology of the sickle cell anemia in India', *The Indian Practitioner* 54 (11): 771-776.

Balgir, R.S. (2005a), 'The spectrum of hemoglobin variant in two scheduled tribes of Sundergarh District in northwestern Orissa, India', *Annals of Human Biology* 32: 560.

Balgir, R.S. (2005b), 'Spectrum of hemoglobinopathies in the state of Orissa in India. A ten-year cohort study. *Journal of the Association of Physicians of India* 53: 1021.

Barsh, G.S., I.S. Farooqi & S. O'Rahilly (2000), 'Genetics of body-weight regulation', *Nature* 404: 644-651.

Basu, S.K. (1994), 'The state of the art of tribal health in India', in S.K. Basu (ed.), *Tribal health in India*. New Delhi: Manak Publication Pvt. Ltd.

Beauman, G., G. Cannon, I. Elmadfa, P. Glasauer, I. Hoffman, M. Keller, M. Krawinkel, T. Lang & C. Leitzman, et al (2005), 'The principles, definition and dimensions of the new nutrition science', *Public Health Nutrition* 8 (6A): 695-698.

Beck, U. (1992), *Risk Society: Towards a new modernity*. London: Sage.

Beck, U. (2007 [1999]), *World Risk Society*. Cambridge: Polity Press.

Beech, H. (2002), 'In rural China, it's a family affair. A dearth of brides has some village bachelors looking for love close to home', *Time* 159 (21) 3 June (Cf. www.time.com/time/asia/magazine/printout/0,13675,501020603-250060,00.html) (Accessed 10 January 2007).

Bell, J. (1998), 'The new genetics in clinical practice', *British Medical Journal* 316: 618-620.

Berg, M. van den, D.R.M. Timmermans & L.P. ten Kate, et al (2005), 'Are pregnant women making informed choices about prenatal screening', *Genetics IN Medicine* 7 (5): 332-338 May/June.

Bonnacorso, M. (2004), 'Programmes of gamete donation: Strategies [private clinics] of assisted conception', in M. Unnithan-Kumar (ed.), *Reproductive agency, medicine and the state: Cultural transformations in childbearing*, 83-102. Oxford: Berghahn.

Borell, B. (2007), First Asian genome sequenced. 12 October. *Nature*. doi:10.1038/news.2007.161.

Brand, A. (2005), 'Public health and genetics – a dangerous combination', *European Journal of Public Health* 15 (2): 113-116 April.

Brandt-Rauf, S. et al (2006), 'Ashkenazi Jews and breast cancer: The consequences of linking ethnic identity to genetic disease', *The American Journal of Public Health* 96 (11): 1979-1988.

Catz, D.S., N.S. Green & J.N. Tobin et al (2005), 'Attitudes about genetics in underserved, culturally diverse populations', *Community Genetics* 8: 161-172.

Cen, Li C. (2004), Zhongguo xingbie bi de xianzhuang ji duoce fenxi fenxi (Analysis on the current situation of sexual proportion of infant in China and the countermeasure)', *Renkou zazhi (Population Journal)* 2: 46-49.

Centers for Disease Control and Prevention (CDC) (2005), 'National vital statistics reports; 54:2'. www.cdc.gov/nchs/data/nvsr/nvsr54/nvsr54_02.pdf.

Cha Byung-hak (2004), 'Bio-tech firm completes draft of Korean genome', *Chosun Ilbo* 26 June. http://kn.koreaherald.co.kr/SITE/data/html_dir/2001/06/30/200106300007.asp [accessed 11.10.03].

Chadwick, R. (2004), 'Nutrigenomics, individualism and public health', *Proceedings of the Nutrition Society* 63: 161-166.

Chan, T.Y. & J.A. Critchley (1996), 'Usage and adverse effects of Chinese herbal medicine', Hum Exp Toxicol 15: 5-12.

Charache, S., M.L. Terrin, R.D. Moore et al (1995), 'Effect of hydroxyurea on the frequency of painful crises in sickle cell anemia', *The New England Journal of Medicine* 332 (20): 1317-1322.

Chee, H.L. & Chan, C.K. (1984), *Designer Genes: I.Q., ideology & biology.* Selangor, Malaysia: Institute for Social Analysis.

Chen, J.-Y. & M.-J Clark (2007), 'Family function in families of children with Duchenne muscular dystrophy', *Family Community Health* 30 (4): 296-304.

Chen, R.-B. & X.-X. Qiu (1999), 'The present status of medical ethics education in the key medical universities in China', in O. Döring (ed.), *Chinese scientists and responsibility. Ethical issues of human genetics in Chinese and international contexts,* 45-55. Hamburg: Mitteilungen des Instituts für Asienkunde 314.

Chen, X. (2005), '*Beijing cheng zhi xujia yilaio guanggao* (Beijing punish medical exaggerated advertisement). *Zhonmghua gongshang bao* (Chinese Industry and Commerce Daily) 8:10.

Chinese Red Cross Foundation (2005), 'Tianshi zhi en' Fund Help 650,000 Children with DMD (taishi zhien jiuzhu 65 wan jijihuaner). www.crcf.org.cn/sys/html/lm_4/2007-09-12/113730.htm.

Chinese Red Cross Foundation (2007), 'Another beneficiary of Tianshi zhien' (tainshi zhien zaici xingdong). www.crcf.org.cn/news/findnews/shownews.asp-newsid=3974.

Chinese Ministry of Health (MOH) (2003), Guidelines for Genetic Counseling (Jiyin Zixun Guifan). www.healthychildren.org.cn/actionplan/fagui/fagui.htm.

Clarke, A.E., L. Mamo, J.R. Fishman, J.K. Shim & J.R. Fosket (2003), 'Biomedicalization: Technoscientific transformations of health, illness, and US biomedicine', *American Sociological Review* 68: 161-194.

Clemens, R & P. Pressman (2004), 'Nutrigenomics: From nutrition to genes', *Food Technology*, 58, 20. www.ift.org/publications/docshop/ft_shop/12-04/12_04_pdfs/12-04-foodmed-health.pdf.

Collins, F.S. (1999), 'Shattuck Lecture – Medical and societal consequences of the Human Genome Project', *The New England Journal of Medicine* 341: 28-37.

Collins, F.S. & V.A. McKusick (2001), 'Implications of the Human Genome Project for medical science', *Journal of the American Medical Association* 285: 540-544.

Council for Science and Technology, Bioethics Committee (2000), *Fundamental principles of research on the human genome.* www.mext.go.jp/a_menu/shinkou/shisaku/fundamen.htm

Council of International Organizations of Medical Sciences (CIOMS) (2002), International ethical guidelines for biomedical research involving human subjects: guidelines 4, 5 and 6.

Critchley, J.A., Y. Zhang, C.C. Suthisisang, T.Y. Chan & B. Tomlinson (2000), 'Alternative therapies and medical science: designing clinical trials of alternative/complementary medicines – is evidence-based traditional Chinese medicine attainable? *Journal of Clinical Pharmacology* 40: 462-7.

Cwik, V. & M. Brooke (1996), 'Disorders of muscle – dystrophies and myopathies', in B. Berg (ed.), *Principles of Child Neurology,* 1665-1671. New York: McGraw-Hill.

Dabrock, P. (2006), 'Public health genetics and social justice', *Community Genetics* 9: 34-39.

Daele, W. van den (2006), 'The spectre of coercion: Is public health genetics the route to policies of enforced disease prevention', *Community Genetics* 9: 40-49.

Daar, A. & P. Singer (2005), 'Pharmacogenetics and geographical ancestry: implications for drug development and global health', *Nature Reviews Genetics* 6: 241-246.

deCastro, L. (2002), 'Reproductive cloning: Moral repugnance and knee-jerk reactions', in Lee Shui-chuen (ed.), Proceedings of the Third International Conference of Bioethics: Ethics, legal and social issues in human pluri-potent stem cell experimentation. Chungli: Central University.

Deok, J.B., K. Jinhyun & W.I. De Silva (2002), 'Induced abortion in Sri Lanka: who goes to providers for pregnancy termination?', *Journal of Biosocial Sciences* 34: 303-315.

Department of Biotechnology, Government of India (DBT) (2002), Ethical policies on human genome, genetic research and services. http://dbtindia.nic.in/policy/ polimain.html

De Silva, D., K.M.S.A.K. Jayasekera, N.K. Rubasinghe & D.G.H. De Silva (1997), 'Attitudes towards genetic counselling and testing among medical students and newly qualified doctors', *Ceylon Medical Journal* 42: 129-132.

De Silva, D., S.C.A. Fisher, A. Premwardhena, S.P. Lambadasuriya, T.E.A. Peto, G. Perera, J.M. Old, J.B. Clegg, N.F. Olivieri, D.J. Weatherall & the Sri Lanka Thalassaemia Group (2000). 'Thalassaemia in Sri Lanka: Implications for the future health burden of Asian populations', *The Lancet* 355: 786-791.

De Soysa, P. (2000), 'Women and health', in S. Jayaweera (ed.), *Post-Beijing Reflections: Women in Sri Lanka 1995-2000'*, Colombo: Centre for Women's Research.

Dikötter, F. (1998), *Imperfect Conceptions*. London: Hurst.

Dissanayake, V.H.W. & R.W. Jayasekara (2008), 'Cytogenetic testing in paediatrics: Some aspects of the Sri Lankan scenario', *Sri Lanka Journal of Paediatrics* 37: 38-41.

Dissanayake, V.H.W., B. Simpson & R.W. Jayasekara (2002), 'Attitudes towards the new genetic and assisted reproductive technologies in Sri Lanka: A preliminary report', *New Genetics and Society* 21 (1): 65-74.

DMD Forum (2001), Guides for Parents-Parenting. www.dmdforum.org/guides/parenting. html.

Döring, O. (1998a), 'Eugenik und Verantwortung: Hintergründe und Auswirkungen des, Gesetzes über die Gesundheitsfürsorge für Mütter und Kinder', *China Aktuell* (08/98): 826-835.

Döring, O. (1998b), 'China and eugenics – preliminary remarks concerning the structure and impact of a problem of international bioethics', *Bioethics in Asia: Proceedings of the UNESCO Asian Bioethics Conference*, 86-91. 3-8 November, Kobe and Fukui, Norio Fujiki & Darryl Macer (eds.) Christchurch: Eubios Ethics Institute.

Döring, O. (ed.) (1999), *Chinese scientists and responsibility. Ethical issues of human genetics in Chinese and international contexts*. Hamburg: Mitteilungen des Instituts für Asienkunde.

Döring, O. (2003a) 'Maßstab im Wandel. Anmerkungen über das Gute und die Medizinethik in China', in Elm, R. & M. Takayama (Hrsg.), *Zukünftiges Menschsein: Ethik zwischen Ost und West*, 319-353. Schriftenreihe des ZEI (Bd. 55), Baden-Baden: Nomos-Verlagsgesellschaft.

Döring, O. (2003b) 'China's struggle for practical regulations in medical ethics', *Nature Reviews Genetics* 4: 233-239.

Döring, O. (2003c), 'Global governance, national state and health system reform: Assessing the case of China', in Hein, W. & L Kohlmorgen (eds.), *Globalization, global health governance and national health politics in developing countries. An exploration into the dynamics of interface*, 269-285. Hamburg: Schriften des Deutschen Übersee-Instituts 60.

Döring, O. (2004), 'Was bedeutet, ethische Verständigung zwischen Kulturen? Ein philosophischer Problemzugang am Beispiel der Auseinandersetzung mit der Forschung an menschlichen Embryonen in China', in Baumann, E., A. Brink, A. May, P. Schröder, & C. Schutzeichel (eds.), 179-212. *Weltanschauliche Offenheit in der Bioethik*, Berlin: Duncker und Humblot.

Döring, O. (2005), 'Der menschliche Embryo in China: Eine Charakterfrage?', in Oduncu, F.S., K. Platzer, W. Henn (Hrsg.), *Der Zugriff auf den Embryo. Ethische, rechtliche und kulturvergleichende Aspekte der Reproduktionsmedizin*, 126-145. Göttingen: Vandenhoek.

Ehara, Y. (1985), Josei kaihō to iu shisō (Thoughts of Women's Liberation). Tokyo: Keisô Shobô.

Ehara, Y. (ed.) (1990), Feminism ronsō – 70 nendai kara 90 nendai e (Feminism Debates: From the 1970s into the 1990s). Tokyo: Keisō Shobō.

Ehara, Y (1991), 'Lib no shuchō to boseikan (The WLM's advocacy and the perspective of motherhood)', in Group lecture on decipherment of motherhood (ed.), Bosei o kaidoku, gedoku suru – Tsukurareta shinwa o koete (Decipherment and antidote of motherhood: Beyond the constructed myth), 194-208. Tokyo: Yūhikaku Sensho no. 799.

Ehara, Y. (1996), Seishokugijutsu to gendā (Reproductive Technology and Gender). Tokyo: Keisô Shobô.

Ehara, Y (1998), 'Feminism mondai e no shôtai (Introduction to feminist issues)', in Ehara, Yumiko (ed.), Feminism no shuchō (Feminist advocacy), 263-310. Tokyo: Keisō Shobō.

Ehara, Y. (2002), Jikoketteiken to gendā (Right to self-determination and gender). Tokyo: Iwanami Shoten.

Elger, B.S. & A.L. Caplan (2006), 'Consent and anonymization in research involving bio-banks', European Molecular Biology Organization Reports 7 (7): 661-666.

Emery, A.E.H. (1991), 'Population frequency of inherited neuromuscular disease – a world survey'. Neuromuscular Disorders 1: 19-29.

Epping-Jordan, J.E., G. Galea, C. Tukuitonga & R. Beaglehole (2005), 'Preventing chronic diseases: Taking stepwise action', The Lancet. Published online 5 October (DOI: 10.1016/S0140-6736(05)67342-4).

Ewing, C.M. (1988), 'Tailored genes: IVF, genetic engineering and eugenics', Reproductive and Genetic Engineering 1 (1): 31-40.

Fan, R.-P. (1997), 'Self-determination vs. family-determination: Two incommensurable principles of autonomy', Bioethics 11 (3&4): 309-322.

Fan, R. (ed.) (1999), Confucian Bioethics. Dordrecht: Kluwer Academic Publishers.

Flood, D.M., N.S. Weiss, L.S. Cook, J.C. Emerson, S.M. Schwartz, J. & D. Potter (2002), 'Colorectal cancer incidence in Asian migrants to the United States and their descendants', Cancer Causes and Control 11 (5): 403-411.

Food Ethics Council (2005), Genetic Personal: Shifting responsibilities for dietary health, December. London: Food Ethics Council.

Foucault, M. (1980), 'Power/knowledge', in C. Gordon (ed.), Selected interviews and other writings 1972-1977. Brighton: Harvester Press.

Foucault, M. (1982), 'The subject and power', in H.L. Dreyfus & P. Rabinow (eds.) Beyond Structuralism and Hermeneutics, 208. Chicago: University of Chicago Press.

Foucault, M. (1991), 'Governmentality', in G. Burchell, G. Colin & P. Miller (eds.) The Foucault Effect Studies in Governmentality, 87-104. London: Harvester Wheatsheaf.

Franklin, S. & C. Roberts (2006), Born and Made. Princeton: Princeton University Press.

Frayling, T.M., N.J. Timpson, M.N. Weedon, E. Zeggini, R.M. Freathy, C.M. Lindgren, J.R. Perry, K.S. Elliott, H. Lango, N.W. Rayner, B. Shields, L.W. Harries, J.C. Barrett, S. Ellard, C.J. Groves, B. Knight, A.M. Patch, A.R. Ness, S. Ebrahim, D.A. Lawlor, S.M. Ring, Y. Ben-Shlomo, M.R. Jarvelin, U. Sovio, A.J. Bennett, D. Melzer, L. Ferrucci, R.J. Loos, I Barroso, N.J. Wareham, F. Karpe, K.R. Owen, L.R. Cardon, M. Walker, G.A. Hitman, C.N. Palmer, A.S. Doney, A.D. Morris, G.D. Smith, A.T. Hattersley, M.I. McCarthy (2007), 'A common variant in the FTO gene is associated with body mass index and predisposes to childhood and adult obesity', Science 11 May; 316 (5826): 889-894. Epub 12 Apr 2007.

Freedman, R., M.-C. Chang & T.-H Sun (1994) 'Taiwan's transition from high fertility to below-replacement levels', Studies in Family Planning 25 (6): 317-331.

Fujii, M. (1993), Sosensaishi no girei kōzō to minzoku (Rituals and folklore of ancestor worship). Kōbundō: Tokyo.

Fujiki, N. (2008), 'Bioethics and medical genetics in Japan', in M. Sleeboom (ed.), Genomics in Asia. London: Routledge.

Fujimura, J.H. (1992), 'Crafting science: standardised packages, boundary objects, and 'translation', in A. Pickering (ed.) *Science Practice and Ordinary Action: Ethnomethodology and Social Studies of Science*, 168-211. Chicago: University of Chicago Press.

Gannett, L. (2001), 'Racism and human genome diversity research: the ethical limits of populational thinking', *Philosophy of Science* 68 (3): S479-S492.

Gao Xiangdong & Xu Yang (2002), 'Ethical issues in the regulation of population growth and reproduction', in Döring & Chen (eds), *Advances in Chinese Medical Ethics. Chinese and International Perspectives*, 327-334. Hamburg (Mitteilungen des Instituts für Asienkunde No.355).

Gardner-Medwin, D. & P. Sharples (1989), 'Some studies of the Duchenne and autosomal recessive types of muscular dystrophy', *Brain Development* 11: 91-97.

Genetic-Medicine-Related Societies (2003), *Guidelines for genetic testing*. http://jshg.jp/pdf/10academies_e.pdf.

Godard, B., S. Raeburn, M. Pembrey, M. Bobrow, P. Farndon & S. Aymé (2003), 'Genetic information and testing in insurance and employment: technical, social and ethical issues', *European Journal of Human Genetics* 11, Suppl. 2: S123-S142.

Goffman, E. (1986), *Stigma: Notes on the management of spoiled identity*, First Touchstone Edition. New York: Simon & Schuster.

Gollust, S.E., S. Chandros Hull & B.S. Wilfond (2002), 'Limitations of direct-to-consumer advertising for clinical genetic testing', *Journal of the American Medical Association* 288 (14): 1762-1767.

Good, B. (1994), *Medicine, Rationality and Experience: An anthropological experience*. Cambridge: Cambridge University Press.

Görman, U. (2006), 'Ethical issues raised by personalized nutrition based on genetic information', *Genes & Nutrition* 1:13-21.

Grayling, A.C. (2005) 'The power to choose a baby's gender', *New Scientist* 2494: 9 April, www.newscientist.com/channel/opinion/mg18624946.700.

Greely, H. (2001), 'Genotype Discrimination: The complex case for some legislative protection', *University of Pennsylvania Law Review* 149: 1483-1505.

Greenhalgh, S. & E.A. Winckler (2005), *Governing China's Population*, 95. Stanford: Stanford University Press.

Gu B.-C. & K. Roy (1995), 'Sex ratio at birth in China, with reference to other areas in Asia: What we know', *Asia-Pacific Population Journal* 10 (3): 17-42.

Gu B.-C. & Y. Xu (1994), 'A comprehensive discussion of the birth gender ratio in China', *Chinese Journal of Population Science* 6 (4): 423.

Gunasekere, P.C. & P.S. Wijesinha (2001), 'Reducing abortions is a public health issue', *Ceylon Medical Journal* 46: 12-14.

Gupta, J.A. (2007), 'Private and public eugenics: genetic testing and screening in India', *Bioethical Inquiry* 4 (3): 217-228.

Hacking, I. (1992), 'The self-vindication of the laboratory sciences', in A. Pickering (ed.) *Science Practice and Ordinary Action: Ethnomethodology and Social Studies of Science*, 29-64. Chicago: University of Chicago Press.

Haga, S.B., M.J. Khoury & W. Burke (2003), 'Genomic profiling to promote a healthy lifestyle: Not ready for prime time', *Nature Genetics* 34: 347-350. http://www.nature.com/ng/journal/v34/n4/full/ng0803-347.html.

Halldenius, L. (2005), 'Dissecting 'discrimination', *Cambridge Quarterly of Healthcare Ethics* 14: 455-463.

Halldenius, L. (2007), 'Genetic discrimination', in M. Hayry, R. Chadwick, V. Arnsaon & G. Arnason (eds), *The ethics and governance of human genetic databases: European perspectives*, 170-180. Cambridge University Press.

Halliday, J. (2007), 'Sciona gains license to explore Asian nutrigenomics potential', *AP-Food Technology.com*. www.ap-foodtechnology.com/news/ng.asp?n=74962-sciona-gtg-person-lised-nutrition-nutrigenomics.

Hanon, H. (2004), 'Early warning. A simple test saves one baby; another falls ill', *The Wall Street Journal*, 17 June.

Harper, P.S. (1988), 'Genetic counseling in Mendelian disorders', in P.S. Harper (ed.), *Practical genetic counselling*, 18-41. London: Wright.

Harper, P.S. (2004), *Practical Genetic Counselling*, 6th edn 100. Oxford: Oxford University Press.

Harris, J. (1997), '"Goodbye Dolly?" – The ethics of human cloning', *Journal of Medical Ethics* 23: 353-360.

Harvey, P. (2000), *An Introduction to Buddhist Ethics*. Cambridge: Cambridge University Press.

Hasegawa, H. (2005), '*Kōdo shōgai hokenkin to jitsumujō no kadai: sekinin kaishikizen hatsubyō no nintei* (Severe disability insurance and issues in practice: defining the onset of illness before the commencement of the period of liability)', *Seimei Hoken Keiei* 73 (1): 99-115.

Hedgecoe, A.M. (2005), 'The politics of personalised medicine: Pharmacogenetics in the clinic', *Cambridge Studies in Society and the Life Sciences*. Cambridge: Cambridge University Press.

Henneman L, Bramsden I, Van Os TAM, et al (2001), 'Attitudes towards reproductive issues and carrier testing among adult patients and parents of children with cystic fibrosis (CF)', *Prenatal Diagnosis* 21: 1-9.

Hjelm M. (1996), 'Ethics of neonatal screening', in S.T. Lam & C.P. Pang (eds), *Neonatal and Perinatal Screening: The Asian Pacific perspective*, 53-55. Hong Kong: The Chinese University of Hong Kong.

Hogarth, S., K. Lidell, T. Ling, S. Sanderson, R. Zimmern & D. Melzer (2007), 'Closing the gaps: enhancing the regulation of genetic tests using responsive regulation', *Food and Drug Law Journal* 62 (4): 831-848.

Holm, S. (2007), 'Should genetic information be disclosed to insurers?', *British Medical Journal* 334: 1196.

Holtzman, N.A. (2006), 'What role for public health in genetics and vice versa', *Community Genetics* 9: 8-20.

Holtzman, N.A. & D. Shapiro (1998), 'The new genetics: Genetic testing and public policy. *British Medical Journal* 316: 852-856.

Hudson, V.M. & A.M. den Boer (2004) *Bare Branches: The security implications of Asia's surplus male population*. Massachusetts: MIT Press.

Human Rights Watch/Asia (1996), *Death by Default: A policy of fatal neglect in China's state orphanages*. New York: Human Rights Watch.

Humphries, S., P.M. Ridker & P.J. Talmud (2004), 'Genetic testing for cardiovascular disease susceptibility: a useful clinical management tool or possible misinformation?', *Arteriosclerosis Thrombosis and Vascular Biology* 24: 628-636.

Ichinokawa, Y. (1996), 'Sei to seishoku o meguru seiji (Politics of sexuality and reproduction)', in Ehara, Y (ed.), *Seishokugijutu to gendā (Reproductive Technology and Gender)*, 163-218. Tokyo: Keisō Shobō.

Ichinokawa, Y. & S. Tateiwa (1998), 'Shōgaisha undō kara miete kuru mono (What are discovered from the movements of people with handicaps)', in *Gendaishisō (Revue de la pensée d'aujourd'hui)*, Seidosha, Tokyo, 26-28: 258-285.

Ichinokawa, Y., S. Kato & A. Tsuge (1996), '*Yuseihogohō wo meguru saikin no doko*' (The recent movement on the eugenic protection law.), in Y. Ehara (ed.), *Seishoku gijutu to gender (New Reproductive Technology and Gender)*, 375-390. Tokyo: Keisō Shobō.

ICMR (2000), *Ethical Guidelines for Biomedical Research on Human Subjects*. New Delhi: Indian Council of Medical Research.

IFSA (Investment and Financial Services Association Limited) (2005), *IFSA standard no. 11.00 'Genetic testing policy'*. www.ifsa.com.au/documents/IFSA%20Standard%20No% 2011.pdf; www.ifsa.com.au/documents/Fact%20Sheet_specialist%20topics_Life%20&% 20Genetics.pdf.

IGD (2005), *IGD forecasts the future of global retailing*. http://www.igd.com/CIR.asp?menuid=50&cirid=1505.

ILSI (2002), 'Concepts of functional foods', *ILSI Europe Concise Monograph Series*. http://europe.ilsi.org/file/ILSIFuncFoods.pdf .

Imanaka, N., K. Kanemura & T. Otsuka (2004), *Private medical insurance in Japan*. www.iaahs2004.de/img/papers/imanaka2.pdf.

Indian Council of Medical Research (ICMR) (2000), Ethical guidelines for biomedical research on human subjects. *ICMR Bulletin* 30 (10): 107-116. Also: http://www.icmr.nic.in/vsicmr/ethical/pdf.

Institute of Food Technologists (undated), *Functional foods: opportunities and challenges*. www.ift.org.

International Huntington Association (IHA) and the World Federation of Neurology Research Group on Huntington's chorea (1994), 'Guidelines for the molecular genetic predictive test in Huntington's disease', *Journal of Medical Genetics* 31 (7): 555-559.

Ishihara, A. (2002), '*Seimei hoken keiyaku to idenshi kensa* (Life insurance contracts and genetic tests)', *Hogaku Seminā* 573: 28-30.

Janssens, A.C. (2006), 'Predictive genetic testing for type 2 diabetes may raise unrealistic expectations', *British Medical Journal* 333: 509-510.

Japan Center for Economic Research (2005), 'Life insurers and the third sector insurance industry', *Japan Financial Report No. 13*. www.jcer.or.jp/eng/pdf/kinyuE13-3.pdf.

Jasanoff, S. (2005), *Designs on Nature: Science and Democracy in Europe and the United States*. Princeton: Princeton University Press.

Jayasekara, R. (1986), 'Acceptance of a genetic service in Sri Lanka: A student viewpoint', *Ceylon Journal of Medical Science* 29: 67-73.

Jayasekara, R. (1989), 'The attitude of doctors and students towards a genetic service in an Asian country: Sri Lanka', *Asia Oceania Journal of Obstetrics and Gynaecology* 15: 267-270.

Jayasekara, R., G.B. Kristl & W. Wertelecki (1988), 'Acceptance of genetic service: A study of physicians in Colombo, Sri Lanka', *Journal of Biosocial Sciences* 20: 1-7

JETRO (Japan External Trade Organization) (2005), 'Ongoing change in Japan's life insurance industry', *Japan Economic Monthly*. www.jetro.go.jp/en/market/report/pdf/2005_48_m.pdf.

Jimmerson, J. (1990), 'Female infanticide in China: An examination of cultural and legal norms', *Pacific Basin Law Journal* 8 (1): 47-79.

Johnson, J.A. & J.L. Bootman (1995), 'Drug-related morbidity and mortality. A cost of illness model', *Archives of Internal Medicine* 155: 1949-1956.

Jonsen, A.R., S.J. Durfy, W. Burke, & A.G. Motulsky (1996), 'The advent of the 'unpatients'', *Nature Medicine* 2 (6): 622-624.

Joost, H.-G., M.J. Gibney, K.D. Cashman, U. Görman, J.E. Hesketh, M. Mueller, B. van Ommen, C.M. Williams & J.C. Mathers (2007), 'Personalised nutrition: status and perspectives', *British Journal of Nutrition* 98: 26-31.

Kant, I. (1996), *Groundwork of the Metaphysics of Morals*. (Cambridge Texts in the History of Philosophy) [translation: Mary J. Gregor], Part 4: 429. Cambridge: Cambridge University Press.

Kaput, J., J.M. Ordovas, L. Ferguson, B. van Ommen, R.L. Rodriguez, L. Allen, B.N. Ames, K. Dawson, B. German, R. Krauss, W. Malyj & M.C. Archer, et al (2005), 'The case for strategic international alliances to harness nutritional genomics for public and personal health', *British Journal of Nutrition* 94: 623-632.

Kate, S.L. (2000), 'Health Problems of Tribal Population Groups from the State of Maharashtra'. http://sickle.bwh.harvard.edu/india_scd.html (Accessed 18/02/2008).

Kate, S.L. & P. Lingojwar (2002), 'Epidemiology of sickle cell disorder in the state of Maharashtra', *International Journal of Human Genetics* 2 (3): 161-167.

Kato, M. (2005), 'Women's rights? Social movements, abortion and eugenics in modern Japan', Ph.D. dissertation at Leiden University, Leiden.

Kato, M. (2007), 'Silence between patients and doctors: the issue of self-determination and amniocentesis in Japan', *Genomics, Society and Policy* 3 (3): 28-42.

Kaur, M. (2005), 'Accreditation and standardisation of labs', *Express Healthcare Management*, November.

Kaye, J. (2006), 'Police collection and access to DNA samples', *Genomics, Society and Policy* 2 (1): 16-72.

Kegley, J. (2004), 'Challenges to informed consent. Challenges to informed consent', *European Molecular Biology Organization reports* 5 (9): 832-836.

Keown, D. (1995), *Buddhism and Bioethics*. Cambridge: Cambridge University Press.

Kerr, A. (2004), *Genetics and Society*. London: Routledge.

Kerr, A. & T. Shakespeare (2002), *Genetic Politics: From eugenics to genome*. Cheltenham: New Clarion Press.

Kim, S., S. Moon & B.M. Popkin (2001), 'Nutrition transition in the Republic of Korea', *Asia Pacific Journal of Clinical Nutrition* 10 (Suppl): S48-S56.

Kimura R. (1993), 'Asian perspectives: Experimentation on human subjects in Japan – bioethical perspectives in a cultural context', in Z. Bankowski, R.J. Levine (eds.), *Ethics and research on human subjects. International guidelines*, 181-187. Geneva: The Council for International Organizations of Medical Sciences (CIOMS).

Kitcher, P. (1996), *The Lives to Come: The genetic revolution and human possibilities*. New York: Simon & Schuster.

Kneller R. (2001), 'Genetic privacy and discrimination', in N. Fujiki, M. Sudo & D. Macer (eds.), *Bioethics and the impact of human genome research in the 21st century*, Eubios Ethics Institute. http://eubios.info/BHGP/BHGP51.htm

Koch, L. & M.N. Svendsen (2005), 'Providing solutions – defining problems: the imperative of disease prevention in genetic counselling', *Social Science & Medicine* 60: 823-832.

Kohrman, M. (1999), 'Grooming *Quezi*: Marriage exclusion and identity formation among disabled men in contemporary China', *American Ethnologist* 26 (4): 890-909.

Konrad, M. (2005), *Narrating the New Predictive Genetics. Ethics, ethnography and science*. Cambridge: Cambridge University Press.

Kumar, N.K., U. Quach & H. Thorsteinsdóttir et al (2004), 'Indian biotechnology – rapidly evolving and industry led', *Nature Biotechnology* 22: 31-36 Supplement December.

Kuo, W. (2008), 'Understanding race at the frontier of pharmaceutical regulation. An analysis of the racial difference debate at the ICH', *Journal of Law, Medicine, and Ethics* 36 (3): 498-505.

Lal A. & M. Kaur (2006), 'Newborn screening for inborn errors of metabolic disorders', chapter presented at the 8th National Conference of the Indian Society for Prenatal Diagnosis and Therapy (ISPAT), New Delhi, 17-19 February 2006. Abstract in *International Journal of Human Genetics*. February (Supplement 2): 42-43.

Lam S.T., C.P. Pang (eds.) (1996), *Neonatal and Perinatal Screening: The Asian Pacific perspectives*. Hong Kong: The Chinese University of Hong Kong.

Lang, T. & M. Heasman (2004), *Food Wars: The global battle for mouths, minds and markets.* London: Earthscan.

Latimer, J. (2007), 'Becoming in-formed: genetic counselling, ambiguity and choice', *Health Care Analysis,* 5 (1): 13-23.

Latz, I. (1981), *Stigma: A social psychological analysis,* 2. Hillsdale: Lawrence Erlbaum Associates.

Laurie, G. (2000), 'Genetics and insurance: Is it "in the public interest" to involve the law?' at the Royal Society, London, 23 October 2000. www.law.ed.ac.uk/ahrc/files/82_lauriegeneticsandinsurancelawoctoo.pdf

Lazarou, J., B.H. Pomeranz, P. N. Corey (1998), 'Incidence of adverse reactions on hospitalized patients. A meta-analysis of prospective studies', *Journal of the American Medical Association* 279: 1200-1205.

Leach-Scully, J., S. Banks & T. Shakespeare (2006), 'Chance, choice and control: Lay debate on pre-natal sex selection', *Social Science and Medicine* 63: 21-31.

Lee, J, C. Campbell & G. Tan, (1992), 'Infanticide and family planning in late Imperial China. The price and population history of rural Liaoning', in Rawski, T.G. & L.M. Li 1992 (eds.), *Chinese History in Economic Perspective,* 145-176. Berkeley: University of California Press.

Lee S.-C. (2002), 'A Confucian assessment of 'personhood'', in O. Döring & R.-B, Chen (eds.) *Advances in Chinese Medical Ethics. Chinese and international perspectives,* 214-222. Hamburg: Mitteilungen des Instituts für Asienkunde 355.

Lee S. (2003), 'Racial profiling of DNA samples: Will it affect scientific knowledge about human genetic variation?', in M. Knoppers (ed.), *Populations and Genetics: Legal and Socio-Ethical Perspectives,* 231-244. Leiden/Boston: Martinus Nijhoff Publishers.

Lee, S. & A. Kleinman (2000), 'Suicide as resistance in Chinese society', in: Perry E.J. & M. Selden (eds.), Chinese society: change, conflict and resistance, 221-240. London: Routledge.

Lemmens, T. (2003), 'Genetics and insurance discrimination: Comparative legislative, regulatory and policy developments and Canadian options', *Health Law Journal:* 41-86.

Lemmens, T., Y. Joly & B. Knoppers (2004), 'Genetics and life insurance: A comparative analysis', *GenEdit* 2 (2): 1-15.

Li, H., Y. Wu, R.J.F. Loos, F.B. Hu, Y. Liu, J. Wang, Z. Yu & X. Lin (2007), 'Variants in FTO gene are not associated with obesity in a Chinese Han population', *Diabetes.* Published online ahead of print 24 October 24 2007 DOI: 10.2337/db07-1130.

Li, L. (1999), 'The feminist approach to bioethics in China', in Döring, O. (ed.) 1999: *Chinese Scientists and Responsibility: Ethical Issues of Human Genetics in Chinese and International Contexts.* Ole Döring (ed.) Mitteilungen des Instituts für Asienkunde Nr. 314, Hamburg, 1999, 161-164.

Li X.-R. (1996), 'Licence to coerce: Violence against women, state responsibility, and legal failures in China's family-planning program', *Yale Journal of Law and Feminism* 8 (1): 145-191.

Lin, T.Y. & M.C. Lin (1980), 'Love, denial and rejection-responses of Chinese families to mental illness', in A. Kleinman & T.Y. Lin (eds.), *Normal and Abnormal Behaviour in Chinese Culture,* 387-401. Boston: D. Reidel.

Lippman, A. (1991), 'Prenatal genetic testing: Constructing needs and reinforcing inequalities', *American Journal of Law and Medicine* 17: 1-2.

Liu, S. (2005), 'Zhongguo de xingbie pianhao (Gender fondness of Chinese couple)', *Renkou Yanjiu (Population Research)* 3: 1-11.

Liu, W., W. Zhao & G.A. Chase (2004), 'Genome scan meta-analysis for hypertension', *American Journal of Hypertension* Dec.; 17 (12 Pt 1): 1100-1106.

Liu, S.L., K.S. Joseph, M.S. Kramer, A. Allen, R. Sauve, I.D. Rusen & S.W. Wen (2002) 'Relationship of prenatal diagnosis and pregnancy termination to overall infant mortality in Canada', *Journal of the American Medical Association* 287 (12): 1561-1567.

Liu, W.W. Zhao & G.A Chase (2004), 'Genome scan meta-analysis for hypertension', *American Journal of Hypertension* Dec; 17 (12 Pt 1): 1100-1106.

Liu, Z. (2006), 'Cultural conception as demonstrated in the choice of medical treatment of Tibetan (Zangmin jiuyi xuanze de wenhua guannian)', *Opening Era (Kaifang Shidai)* 4: 111-123.

Lock, M. (1980) *East Asian Medicine in Urban Japan: Varieties of Medical Experience.* Berkeley: University of California Press.

Lock, M. (2005), 'Eclipse of the gene and the return of divination', *Current Anthropology* 46 (Supplement): 47-71.

Macer, D. (2003), 'Genetic information in the family in Japan', in D. Cooper (ed.), *Encyclopaedia of the Human Genome,* 855-859. Nature MacMillan. www.eubios.info/Papers/nate587. htm.

Macer, D. & M.A. Chen Ng, (2000), 'Changing attitudes to biotechnology in Japan', *Nature Biotechnology* 18: 945-947.

McGleenan, T. (2000), 'Legal and policy issues in genetics and insurance', *Community Genetics* 3: 45-49.

Mackenzie, C. & N. Stoljar (2000), *Relational Autonomy: Feminist perspectives on autonomy, agency and the social self.* Oxford: Oxford University Press.

Macrogen, Inc. www.macrogen.com/english/index.html (accessed 11/10/03).

Manson, N.C. & O. O'Neill (2007), *Rethinking Informed Consent in Bioethics.* Cambridge: Cambridge University Press.

Mao, X. (1998), 'Chinese geneticists' view of ethical issues in genetic testing and screening: Evidence for eugenics in China', *American Journal of Human Genetics* 63: 688-695.

Mao, X. & D. Wertz (1997), 'China's genetics services provider's attitudes towards several ethical issues: A cross-cultural survey', *Clinical Genetics* 52: 100-109.

Marchand, L.L. (1999), 'Combined influence of genetic and dietary factors on colorectal cancer incidence in Japanese Americans', *Journal of the National Cancer Institute. Monographs* 26: 101-105.

Markman, M. (2004), 'Genetic discrimination arising from cancer risk assessments: a societal dilemma', *Cleveland Clinic Journal of Medicine* 71 (1): 12-18.

Marteau, T.M. & M. Johnston (1986), 'Determinants of beliefs about illness: a study of parents of children with diabetes, asthma, epilepsy, and no chronic illness', *Journal of Psychosomatic Research* 30: 673-683.

Martin, P. et al (2006), *False Positive? Prospects for the clinical and commercial development of pharmacogenetics.* Nottingham: University of Nottingham/University of York.

Masson, L.F., G. McNeill & A. Avenell (2002), 'Genetic variation and the lipid response to dietary intervention: a systematic review', *American Journal of Clinical Nutrition* 77: 1098-1011.

Masson, L.F. & G. McNeill (2005), 'The effect of genetic variation on lipid response to dietary change: Recent findings', *Current Opinion in Lipidology* 16 (1): 61-67.

Matsubara, Y. (2002), '*Botai hogohou no rekishiteki haikei*' (The historical background of the maternal protection law), in Y. Saito (ed.), *Botaihogoho to Watashitati (The maternal body protection law and us)*, 35-48. Tokyo: Akashi Shoten.

Matsuda, I. (2003), 'Genetic health care services, present and near future in Japan', *Eubios Journal of Asian and International Bioethics* 13: 57-58.

Matsuda, I. (2004), 'Japan', in D. Wertz and J. Fletcher (eds.), *Genetics and Ethics in Global Perspective*, 251-261. Dordrecht: Kluwer.

Mayor, S. (2005), 'UK insurers postpone using predictive testing until 2011', *British Medical Journal* 330: 617.

Mehl, B. & J. Santell (2000), 'Projecting future drug expenditures', *American Journal of Health System Pharmacy* 57 (2): 129-138.

Mehrotra, I. (2004), 'A perspective on developing and marketing food products to meet individual needs of population segments', *Comprehensive Reviews in Food Science and Food Safety* 3: 142-144.

Meijboom, F.L.B., M.F. Verweij & F.W.A. Brom (2003), 'You eat what you are: Moral dimensions of diets tailored to one's genes', *Journal of Agricultural and Environmental Ethics* 16: 557-568.

Mittra, J. (2007), 'Predictive genetic information and access to life assurance: the poverty of 'genetic exceptionalism'', *BioSocieties* 2: 349-373.

Miyachi, T. (2000), '*Idenshi jyohō to seimeihoken jigyō* (Genetic information and the life insurance industry)', *Bunkenronshū* 131: 225-275.

Miyachi, T. (2004) '*Hokengaku o kenkyu shite omō koto* (Thoughts on the study of insurance)', *Access FSA* 18: 14-18. www.fsa.go.jp/access/16/200405.pdf

Miyachi, T. (2005), '*Idenshi kensa to hoken* (The impact of genetic testing on insurance)', *Financial Services Agency Research Review*. www.fsa.go.jp/frtc/nenpou/2005/06.pdf

Montoya, M.J. (2007), 'Bioethnic conscription: Genes, race, and mexicana/o ethnicity in diabetes research', *Cultural Anthropology* 22 (1): 94-128.

Morioka M. (2004), 'Cross-cultural approaches to the philosophy of life in the contemporary world: From bioethics to life studies', in M. Sleeboom (ed.), *Genomics in Asia*, Chapter 10. London: Routledge.

Morrison, P.J. (2005), 'Insurance, unfair discrimination, and genetic testing', *Lancet* 366: 877-880.

Munro, D. (ed.) (1985), *Individualism and Holism: Studies in Confucian and Taoist values*. Ann Arbor, Center for Chinese Studies: University of Michigan Press.

Munro, D. (1988), *Images of Human Nature. A Sung Portrait*. Princeton: Princeton University Press.

Murata, T. (2001), '*Minkan seimeihoken no shikumi* (The structure of private life insurance)', *Hokengakuzasshi* 574: 36-46.

Mutō, K. (2000), *Gyaku sentaku no bōshi to "shiranai de iru kenri" no kakuho: Igirisu no han-chintonbyou idenshikensa kekka wo tegakari ni* (Securing the prevention of adverse selection and "the right not to know": Lessons from the commercial use of Huntington's disease test results in the UK). http://homepage1.nifty.com/JHDN/pdfs/hdukadvslc.pdf .

Murray, R.D. (2002), 'Historical perspective: The sickle cell testing debacle', *J Minority Med Stud.* (spec suppl.) *Human Genome Project Black Bag* [serial online]. Also: www.ornl.gov/sci/techresources/Human_Genome/publicat/jmmbbag.pdf (Accessed on 29/11/2004).

Nagaraja, S.M., S. Jain & U.B. Muthane (2006), 'Perspectives towards predictive testing in Huntington disease', *Neurology India* 54 (4): 359-362.

NASTEC (2003), *New genetics and assisted reproductive technologies in Sri Lanka: a draft national policy on biomedical ethics*. Colombo: National Science and Technology Commission (doc ref NSTC-SG-09/03/01).

National Human Genome Research Institute (2001), 'Developing a haplotype map of the human genome for genes related to health and disease.' July 18-19. Available at: www.genome.gov/10001665.

National Human Genome Research Institute (2002), 'International HapMap Project.' October. Available at: www.genome.gov/10005340.

Nestle, M. (2002), *Food Politics*. Berkeley: University of California Press.

Newborn Screener (2005), A Quarterly Newsletter on Inborn Errors of Metabolism, 1(1), May.

Nie J.-B. (2000), "'So bitter that no word can describe it'": Mainland Chinese women's experience and narratives of abortion', in Tang, R. (ed.), *Globalizing Feminist Bioethics: Women's health concerns worldwide*, 190-211. Boulder & London: Westview Press.

Nie, Jing-Bao (2005), *Behind the Silence. Chinese voices on abortion.* Lanham & Oxford: Rowman & Littlefield.

NIPSSR (National Institute of Population and Social Security Research) (2007), *Social security in Japan.* www.ipss.go.jp/s-info/e/Jasos2007/SS2007.pdf.

Nishinihon Shinbun, (2008), 'Senshokukutai ijō no chōonpakensa no sonzai ishi, oshieru gimunashi sankaidantai ga hatsushishin (Medical doctors have no obligation to tell their patients that ultrasound can detect chromosomal disorders)'. 31 March.

Nordgren, A. (2001), *Responsible Genetics: The moral responsibility of geneticists for the consequences of genetic research.* Amsterdam: Springer.

Norgren, T. (2001), *Abortion before Birth Control: The politics of reproduction in Postwar Japan.* New Jersey: Princeton University Press.

Novas, P. & N. Rose (2000), 'Genetic risk and the birth of the somatic individual', *Economy and Society* 29 (4): 485-513.

Ogino, M. (2004), 'Reproductive technologies and the feminist dilemma in Japan', paper presented at the conference, 'Going too far: Rationalizing unethical medical research in Japan, Germany, and the United States', at the University of Pennsylvania, Philadelphia, 29 April.

Okada, T. (2001), '*Idenshi shindan to hokengyō no hōteki kōsaku* (Legal relationship between genetic test and insurance business)', *Hokengaku Zasshi* 574: 62-86.

O'Neill, O. (1998), 'Insurance and genetics: the current state of play', in R. Brownsword, W.R. Cornish & M. Llewelyn (eds.), *Law and Human Genetics: Regulating a revolution*, 124-131. Oxford: Hart.

Otomo, T. (2005), *The growth of private medical insurance market in Japan.* http://www.actuaries.org/EVENTS/Seminars/EAAC_Bali/16%20(286-306)%20Takahito_Otomo.pdf .

Ozasa, Y. (2006), 'Yōsuikensa, iryôgenba deno shien (Amniocentesis: Support at the medical practice)', in Post-genomic jidai ni okeru seibutsu-igaku to gender 'ikagaku gijutsu ni okeru literacy o kangaeru, Ochanomizu University the 21st Century COE Programme, Frontiers of Gender Studies series 19, 76-85.

Paradies, Y.C., M.J. Montoya & S.M. Fullerton (2007), 'Racialized genetics and the study of complex diseases', *Perspectives in Biology and Medicine* 50 (2): 203-227.

Parsons, E.P., A.J. Clarke, K. Hood & D.M. Bradley (2000), 'Feasibility of a change in service delivery: The case of optional newborn screening for Duchenne muscular dystrophy', *Community Genetics* 3:17-23.

Patra, P.K. & M. Sleeboom-Faulkner (2007a), 'Informed consent and benefit sharing in genetic research and biobanking in India: an anthropological perspective'. Paper presented at the International Conference for Junior Researchers on 'Justice, Fairness and Biobanking – Conflicting Concepts? Ethical, legal and social perspectives regarding the claims for personal integrity, social obligation and sharing of benefits', 8-14 October 2007 at Phillipps-University of Marburg, Germany.

Patra, P.K. & M. Sleeboom-Faulkner (2007b), 'Genetic biobanking in India – a community based perspective on ways and means of data generation', *Taiwan Journal of Law and Technology Policy* 4 (1): 67-97.

Patra, P.K. & M. Sleeboom-Faulkner (2008), 'The Indian genomic biobank initiative and emerging bioethical issues: A community based perspective', in M. Sleeboom-Faulkner (ed.), *Human Genetic Biobanks in Asia: Politics of trust and scientific advancement.* London & New York: Routledge.

Paul, G. (1996), 'Philosophie. Die Ontologisierung der Ethik, Tradition, Moderne und Humanität', in Mall, R.A. & N. Schneider (eds.), *Studien zur interkulturellen Philosophie* Bd. 5, 183-197. Amsterdam: Rodopi.

Pearce, N. (1996), 'Traditional epidemiology, modern epidemiology, and public health', *American Journal of Public Health* 86: 678-683.

Perera, A.C. (2006), 'Testing the mushrooming medical tests', www.srilankahr.net/modules. php?name=Content&pa=showpage&pid=154&cid (accessed 28 June 2006).

Petersen, A. (1998), 'The new genetics and the politics of public health', *Critical Public Health* 8: 59-71.

Petersen, A. (2003), 'The new genetics and citizenship', LSE Vital Politics conference, London 6-7 Sep. www.lse.ac.uk/collections/BIOS/vital_politics_papers.htm.

Petersen, A. (2006), 'The genetic conception of health: is it as radical as claimed?', *Health* 10 (4): 481-500.

Peverelli, P. (2001), 'China and the West: Can we learn from each other?', *Functional Ingredients* Sept-Oct. www.ffnmag.com/ASP/articleDisplay.asp?strArticleId=239&strSite=FFNSite.

Phillips, M., H.-Q. Liu & Y.-P. Zhang (1999), 'Suicide and social change in China', *Culture Med Psychiatry* 23: 25-50.

Popkin, B.M. & P. Gordon-Larsen, (2004), 'The nutrition transition: Worldwide obesity dynamics and their determinants', *International Journal of Obesity* 28: S2-S9.

Prainsack B. & G. Siegal (2006), 'The rise of genetic couplehood? A comparative view of premarital genetic testing', *Biosocieties* 1: 17-36.

Qiu, J. & E. Hayden (2008), 'Genomics sizes up', *Nature* 16 January 451: 234. doi:10.1038/451234a.

Qiu R.-Z. (2000), 'Reshaping the concept of personhood: A Chinese perspective', in Becker, G.K. (ed.), *The Moral Status of Persons: Perspective on bioethics.* Amsterdam & Atlanta: Rodopi.

Qiu R.-Z. (2003), 'Cloning in biomedical research and reproduction: ethical and legal constraints – a Chinese perspective', in Honnefelder, L. & D. Lanzerath (eds.), *Cloning in Biomedical Research and Reproduction. Scientific aspects – ethical, legal and social limits,* 667-678. Bonn: Bonn University Press.

Qiu, R.-Z. (ed.) (2006), *Bioethics: Asian perspectives. A quest for moral diversity.* Dordrecht: Kluwer.

Ragothaman, M. et al (2006), 'Direct costs of managing Parkinson's disease in India: Concerns in a developing country', *Movement Disorders* 21 (10): 1755-1758.

Ramseyer, J.M. (2007), 'Talent and expertise under universal health insurance: The case of cosmetic surgery in Japan', *Discussion Paper No. 600.* www.law.harvard.edu/programs/olin_center/papers/pdf/Ramseyer_600.pdf.

Rapp, R. (1999), *Testing Women, Testing the Fetus: The social impact of amniocentesis in America.* New York and London: Routledge.

Raz, A.E. & M. Atar (2004), 'Upright generations of the future – tradition and medicalization in community genetics', *Journal of Contemporary Ethnography* 33 (3): 296-322.

Roetz, H. (1993), *Confucian Ethics of the Axial Age.* New York: SUNY Press.

Roetz, H. (2004), 'On nature and culture in Zhou China', in Dux, G. & H.U. Vogel (eds.), *Concepts of Nature in Traditional China: Comparative approaches,* Leiden: Brill.

Rohlen, T.P. (1974), 'Entrance, departure, and 'lifelong commitment'', in *For Harmony and Strength.* Berkeley: University of California Press.

Rose, H. (2003), 'An ethical dilemma: the rise and fall of UmanGenomics – the model biotech company?', *Nature* 425: 123-124.

Rosenberg, N. et al (2002), 'Genetic substructure of humans', *Science* 298 (5602): 2381-2385.

Rosmond, R. (2003), 'Association studies of genetic polymorphisms in central obesity: A critical review', *International Journal of Obesity* 27: 1141-1151.

Rothenberg, K.H. & E.J. Thomson (eds.) (1994), *Women and Prenatal Testing: Facing the challenges of genetic technology*. Columbus: Ohio State University Press.

Rothman, B.K. (1993), *The Tentative Pregnancy: How amniocentesis changes the experience of motherhood*. London; W.W. Norton & Company.

Rubin, S. (1987), 'The psychological impact of genetic disease', in L. Charash, R. Lovelace, S. Wolf, A. Kutscher, D. Roye & C. Leach (eds), *Realities in Coping with Progressive Neuromuscular Diseases*, 209-215. Philadelphia: The Charles Press.

Ryder, S. (2005), 'Scientists create Japan's largest biobank for genetic studies of 47 common diseases', *Affymetrix Microarray Bulletin*. www.microarraybulletin.com/community/article.php?p=32.

Sagou, H., T. Okuyama & H. Kawane (2002), '*Shusanki Iden Counseling System Kōchiku ni kansuru Kenkyu: Sanka Iryo ni okeru Iden Counseling*' (A study for establishing perinatal counselling system: A genetic counselling in gynaecology) in J. Furuyama (ed.), *Iden Counseling Taisei no Kōchiku ni kansuru Kenkyu. Kousei-roudou Kagaku Kenkyu (Research-in-aid by Minister of Health and Labor)*, 629-641. Tokyo: Kousei-roudou sho (Ministry of Health, Welfare and Labor).

Saitô, Y. (ed.) (2002) *Botaihogoho to watashitachi – Chūzetsu, tatai gensū, funinshujutsu wo meguru seido to watashitachi (The Law to Protect Mothers' Bodies and us: The system around abortion, the operation of multiple pregnancy and sterilisation, and society)*. Tokyo: Akashi Shoten.

Sander, C. (2000), 'Genomic medicine and the future of health care', *Science* 287: 1977-1978.

Sartorius, N. (1997) 'Fighting schizophrenia and its stigma', A New World Psychiatric Association Educational Programme. *British Journal of Psychiatry* 170: 297.

Sato, K. (1999), *Shusseizen Shindan: Inochi no Hinshitsu Kanri eno Keisho (Prenatal diagnosis: warning against quality control of life)* Tokyo: Yuhikaku.

Savulescu, J. (1999a), 'Sex selection: the case for', *Medical Journal of Australia* 171: 373-375.

Savulescu, J. (1999b), 'Should doctors intentionally do less then the best?', *Journal of Medical Ethics* 25(2): 121-126. April.

Saxena, R. (2006), 'Prenatal diagnosis of hemoglobinopathies in India', chapter presented at the 8th National Conference of the Indian Society for Prenatal Diagnosis and Therapy (IS-PAT), New Delhi, 17-19 February 2006. Abstract in *International Journal of Human Genetics*. February (Supplement 2): 36.

Scharping T. (2003), *Birth Control in China 1949-2000. Population policy and demographic development*. London. New York: RoutlegeCurzon.

Schatz, H. & M. Pfohl (2001), 'Strategies for the prevention of type 2 diabetes', *Experimental and Clinical Endocrinology and Diabetes*, 109 (Suppl. 2): S240-S249.

Sentensei shishi shôgai ji fubo no kai, ed., *Korega bokurano gotai manzoku (This is our perfect bodies)*, Sanseidô, Tokyo, 1999.

Siegelman, P. (2004), 'Adverse selection in insurance markets: an exaggerated threat', *The Yale Law Journal* 113:1223-1281.

Silver, L.M. (1999), *Remaking Eden. Cloning, Genetic Engineering and the Future of Humankind?* London: Phoenix.

Simpson, B. (2001), 'Ethical regulation and the new reproductive technologies in Sri Lanka: the perspectives of ethics committee members', *Ceylon Medical Journal* 46 (2): 54-57.

Simpson, B. (2007), 'On parrots and thorns: Sri Lankan perspectives on genetics, science and the concept of personhood', *Health Care Analysis* 15 (1): 41-49.

Simpson, B., V.H.W. Dissanayake, D. Wickremasinghe & R.W. Jayasekera (2003), 'Prenatal testing and pregnancy termination in Sri Lanka: the views of doctors and medical students', *Ceylon Medical Journal* 48 (4): 129-132.

Simpson, B., V.H.W. Dissanayake & R.W. Jayasekera (2005), 'Contemplating choice: attitudes towards intervening in reproduction in Sri Lanka', *New Genetics and Society* 24 (1): 99-118.

Singer, P. & A.S. Daar (2001), 'Harnessing genomics and biotechnology to improve global health equity', *Science* 294 (5540): 87-89.

Sleeboom-Faulkner, M. (ed.) (2004a), *Genomics in Asia: Cultural values and bioethical practices*. London: Kegan Paul.

Sleeboom-Faulkner, M. (2004b), 'Socio-genetic marginalization in Asia. A plea for a comparative approach to the relationship between genomics, governance, and social-genetic identity', in G. Árnason, S. Nordal & V. Árnason (eds), *Blood and data. Ethical, legal and social aspects of human genetic databases*, 39-44. Reykjavík: University of Iceland Press.

Sleeboom-Faulkner, M. (2006), 'How to define a population: Cultural politics of genetic sampling in the People's Republic of China (PRC) and the Republic of China (ROC)', *Biosocieties* December; 1 (4): 399-420.

Smedley, B., A. Stith, & A. Nelson (2002), 'Unequal Treatment: Confronting Racial and Ethnic Disparities in Health Care', Institute of Medicine of the Academics of Medicine. 20 March.

Stafford, C. (1995), *The Roads of Chinese Childhood: Learning and identification in Angang*. Cambridge: Cambridge University Press.

Steinberg, N., F. Barton, O. Castro et al (2003), 'Effect of hydroxyurea on mortality and morbidity in adult sickle cell anemia', *Journal of the American Medical Association* 289 (13): 1645-1651.

Stock, G. (2002), *Redesigning Humans. Choosing Our Children's Genes*. London: Profile Books.

Stuart, C. (2000), 'Human genetic databases in Japan', UK Parliament Select Committee on Science and Technology, Memorandum by the Science and Technology Section of the British Embassy, Tokyo. www.publications.parliament.uk/pa/ld199900/ldselect/ldsctech/115/115we10.htm.

Sugano, S. (2001), 'Pregnant women's attitude on having prenatal diagnosis and practitioners' participation', in *Hoken iryō shakaigaku ronshū* 12: 115-126.

Sugiyama-Lebra, T. (1984), *Japanese Women: Constraint and fulfillment*. Honolulu: University of Hawaii Press.

Sui, S. & M. Sleeboom-Faulkner (2007), 'Commercial genetic testing in Mainland China: Social, financial and ethical issues', *Journal of Bioethical Inquiry* December 4 (3): 229-237.

Sung, W.-C. (2008), 'Within borders: Risks and the development of biobanking in China', in M. Sleeboom-Faulkner (ed.) *Human Genetic Biobanks in Asia: Politics of trust and scientific advancement*, Ch. 9. London: Routledge.

Suzuki, R. (2005), 'Private health care insurance: Shouldering risk at the individual level', *JCER Research Report 58*. www.jcer.or.jp/eng/pdf/kenrepo50407e.pdf.

Swann, N.L. (1932), *Pan Chao: Foremost woman scholar of China*. New York: Century.

Taioli, E & S. Garte (2002), 'Covariates and confounding in epidemiologic studies using metabolic gene polymorphisms', *International Journal of Cancer* 100: 97-100.

Takamune, I. (1972), *Josei no rekishi (The History of Women)*, vol. 2, Tokyo: Kōdansha.

Takebe, H. (2002), 'Hitogenomu ni miru kōshi mondai (Public private issues in the human genome project)', in S. Tsuyoshi & K.T. Chang (eds.), *Kagakugijutsu to kōkyōsei, Tokyo: Daigaku Shuppankai*.

Takeda, C. (1957), *Senzo sūhai (Ancestor Worship)*. Kyoto: Heirakuji Shoten.

Tanaka, M. (1973), 'Matamata yuseihogoho kaiaku nanoda!: shogaisha mondai wo chushin ni' (Resist the movement for corrupting the eugenic protection law again: thinking about the issues on disabled people), *Lib News* 3: 1-4.

Tarr, J. (2002), 'Regulatory approaches to genetic testing in insurance', *Sydney Law Review* 24 (2): 189-206.

T'ein J.-K. (1988), *Male Anxiety and Female Chastity: A comparative study of Chinese ethical values in Ming-Ch'ing times*, 28-30. Leiden: Brill.

Thakore, D. (1994), 'Thalassemia's bloody battle', *The Times of India*, 27 February 1994.

Thomas R.G. (2007), 'Effect on premiums is small', *British Medical Journal* 334: 1288.

TIHF/GAH Sickle Cell Disease Center Nilgiri District, South India (2007), www.tihf.org/scd.htm.

Tremain, S. (2006), 'Reproductive freedom, self-regulation, and the government of impairment in utero', *Hypatia* 21 (1): 35-53.

Tsuge, A., S. Sugano & M. Ishiguro (2005), The Comparative Study of Women's Decision-Making Processes in Prenatal Tests, A Report for Grant-in-Aid for Scientific Research by the Japan Society for the Promotion of Sciences (Class C).

Tsuji, K. (2003), 'Women's experiences of subsequent pregnancy and childbirth following delivery of a child with Down's syndrome', *Journal of Japan Academy of Nursing Science* 23 (1): 46-56.

Tsukamoto, Y. (2005), *Iryo no naka no ishi kettei – Shusseizenshindan (Self-determination in medicine: Prenatal diagnosis)*, Kouchishobo. Tokyo: Kōchi shobō.

UNICEF (2004) The Official Summary of the State of the World's Children. New York: UNICEF.

United Nations University (1993), The Impact of Economic Development on Rural Women in China. Tokyo: United Nations University.

United States Government Accountability Office (2006), Nutrigenetic testing: Tests purchased from four sites mislead consumers. July. www.gao.gov/new.items/d06977t.pdf.

Unnithan, M. (ed.) (2006), Reproductive Agency, Medicine and the State. New York & Oxford: Berghahn Books.

Urtizberea, J.A., Q.-S. Fanb, E. Vroom, D. Re'can & J.-C. Kaplan (2003), 'Looking under every rock: Duchenne muscular dystrophy and traditional Chinese medicine', Neuromuscular Disorders 13: 705-707.

USNIH (United States National Institutes of Health), National Cancer Institute (2006), Probability of breast cancer in American women. www.cancer.gov/cancertopics/factsheet/Detection/probability-breast-cancer.

Verma, I.C. & S. Bijarnia (2002), 'The burden of genetic disorders in India and a framework for community control', *Community Genetics* 5: 192-196.

Verma, I.C., R. Saxena, M. Lall, S. Bijarnia & R. Sharma (2003), 'Genetic counselling and prenatal diagnosis in India – experience at Sir Ganga Ram Hospital', *Indian Journal of Pediatrics* 70 (4): 293-297.

Vineis, P & D.C. Christiani (2004), 'Genetic testing for sale', *Epidemiology* 15 (1): 3-5.

Vineis, P., H. Ahsan & M. Parker (2005), 'Genetic screening and occupational and environmental exposures', *Journal of Occupational and Environmental Medicine* 62: 657-662.

Wade, P. (2002), Race, Nature and Culture. An Anthropological Perspective. London: Pluto Press.

Wahlqvist, M.L., G. Savige & N. Wattanapenpaiboon (2004), 'Cuisine and health: A new initiative for science and technology – "The Zhejiang Report" from Hangzhou', Asia Pacific Journal of Clinical Nutrition 13 (2): 121-124.

Wallace, H.M. (2005a), 'Who regulates genetic tests?', Nature Reviews Genetics 6 (7): 517.

Wallace, H.M. (2005b), 'Genetic testing and insurance', The Biochemist 27 (4): 37-39.

Wallace, H.M. (2006a), 'Your diet tailored to your genes: Preventing diseases or misleading marketing?', GeneWatch UK. www.genewatch.org.

Wallace, H.M. (2006b), 'Diet-related disease: Nutrigenomics: The solution?', AgroFood Industry Hi-Tech 17 (4): July/August 2006.

Wallace, H.M. (2006c), 'A model of gene-gene and gene-environment interactions and its implications for targeting environmental interventions by genotype', Theoretical Biology and Medical Modeling 3:35. www.tbiomed.com/content/3/1/35.

Waldschmidt, A. (1992), 'Against selection of human life: People with disabilities oppose genetic counseling', Issues in Reproductive and Genetic Engineering 5: 2155-2167.

Walsh, D. & D. Li (2004), 'The food industry and provincial economies', Asia Pacific Journal of Clinical Nutrition 13 (2): 166-170.

Wang, K.W.K. & A. Barnard (2004), 'Technology-dependent children and their families: A review. Journal of Advanced Nursing 45: 36-46.

Wang, S. & S.K. Zhang (2002), Jibing de wenhua yinyue (The cultural metaphor of disease). Yixue yu zhexue (Medicine and Philosophy) 9: 22-25.

Watanabe, A. & T. Shimada, (2005), 'Igakubugakusei o taishō to shita rinshōiden ni kansuru rikaidochōsa – Igakubu ni okeru rinshōidenkyōiku no hitsuyōsei (A questionnaire study of medical students' comprehension of clinical genetics: The Necessity of education in clinical genetics in medical school)', Igaku kyōiku 36:4.

Watson, R. & P.B. Ebrey (1991), Marriage and Inequality in Chinese Society. Berkeley: University of California Press.

Weatherall, D. & J.B. Clegg (2001), The Thalassaemia Syndromes. Oxford: Blackwell Science.

Weedon, M.N., M.I. McCarthy, G. Hitman, M. Walker, C.J. Groves, E. Zeggini, N.W. Rayner, B. Shields, K.R. Owen, A.T. Hattersley & T.M. Frayling (2006), 'Combining information from common type 2 diabetes risk polymorphisms improves disease prediction', PloS Medicine 3 (10): e374.

Wertz, D.C., J.C. Fletcher & K. Berg (2003), Review of ethical issues in medical genetics. Report of consultants to WHO. Geneva: World Health Organization Human Genetics Programme.

Wilkie, D. (1997), 'Mutuality and solidarity: assessing risks and sharing', Philosophical Transactions: Biological Sciences 352 (1357): 1039-1044.

World Health Organization (WHO) (1998), Proposed international guidelines on ethical issues in medical genetics and genetics services, Section 6.

World Health Organization (WHO) (2002), Genomics and world health: report of the advisory committee on health research. Geneva: World Health Organization.

World Health Organization (2003), 'Diet, nutrition and the prevention of chronic diseases. Report of a joint WHO/FAO expert consultation', WHO Technical Report Series: 916.

Wu, Y. (2007), 'Discrimination rife against carriers of hepatitis virus', China Daily, 23 March.

Xie, H-G, et al (2001), 'Molecular basis in ethnic differences in drug disposition and response', Annual Review of Pharmacology and Toxicology 41: 815-850.

Xinhuanet (2003), 'First national family planning law highlights humanitarianism', 24 November, http://www.chinaembassy.org.au/eng/xw/t45746.htm.

Xinran (2003), The Good Women of China. London: Vintage.

Yamashita, N. (2004), 'Kōdo shōgai hokenkin seikyūken no shiharai yōken ha jūsoku shiteinai to shinagara mo hokenkaisha no shibuchō no taiō nado kara kōdo shōgai hokenkin no shiharai o kyohi suru koto ha shingisoku ihan ni gaitō suru toshite shiharai o ninyō shita jirei (A case where the conditions for payment of insurance money under a severe disability policy were not met but, due to the branch office manager's actions, the refusal of payment of the insurance money was held to violate the duty to act in good faith)', Kinyū Shōji Hanrei 1198 (1): 62-68.

Yang, J. (2008), 'The power relationships between doctors, patients and the party-state under the impact of red packets in the Chinese health-care system', PhD dissertation, School of Social Sciences and International Studies, University of New South Wales.

Ye T.-X. (2003), Throwaway Daughter. New York: Doubleday.

Yokota, H. (2004), Hiteisareru inochi karano toi: Nôsei mahi sha to shite ikite (Questions raised by a denied life: Living as a person with CP). Tokyo: Gendai Shokan.

Yokota, H. & T. Yonezu (2004), 'Yūsei shisō, shōgai, josei no sei to seishoku no kenri (Eugenic thoughts, handicaps and women's sexual and reproductive rights)', in H. Yokota (ed.), Hiteisareru inochi karano toi: Nōsei mahi sha to shite ikite (Questions raised by a denied life: Living as a person with CP), 67-123. Tokyo: Gendai Shokan.

Yonezu, T. (2002), 'Shogaisha to Josei: Renndo-shi Hokan-shiau Sabetsu soshite Kaiho' (Disabled people and women: thinking about discrimination and liberation), SOSHIREN News 204: 10-21.

Yoshizumi, K. (1995), 'Marriage and family: Past and present', in K. Fujimura-Fanselow & A. Kameda. (eds.), Japanese Women, 183-198. New York: The Feminist.

Yuan, T.H. (1991), China's Strategic Demographic Initiative. New York: Praeger.

Yûseihogohô kaiaku soshi renrakukai (Soshiren) et al (1996), Mou iranai! Dataizai to yûsehogo – Watashi no karada, watashiga kimeru (No need for abortion criminal law, the Eugenic Protection Law: My body, I decide), Tokyo, 1996. (A summary and materials of activity, meeting report from a symposium held on February 24, 1996, in Tokyo.)

Zeggini, E. & M.I. McCarthy (2007), 'TCF7L2: the biggest story in diabetes genetics since HLA', Diabetologia 50: 1-4.

Zhang, X. (2005) Tianshi zhi En Jijin jianli (Kindness from angel; Fund established). Guangming Ribao (Guangming Daily). 11: 17.

Zheng, A., Y. Wen & R. MacLennan (2004), 'Cuisine: The concept and its health and nutrition implications – a Hangzhou perspective', Asia Pacific Journal of Clinical Nutrition 13 (2): 136-140.

Zheng, Z. (2004), Zhongguo yihun funiu de shnegyu yuanwang (Fertility desire of married women in China)', Zhongguo renkou kexue (Chinese Journal of Population Science) 5: 73-78.

Website

www.dbtindia.nic.in/programmes/progmain.html (accessed: 14 July 2006 and 5 March 2007).

Index

'ability to perform one's role' 138
abortion 32, 92, 109, 111, 113, 116
– attitudes to in Japan 112
– choice 224
– coercion 225
– Japan 113
– sex selection (China) 197
– sex selective 189, 192
– sex-selection 194
access to basic knowledge 167
access to facilities 76
access to healthcare 87
access to technology 79
access to testing
– distribution 80
– expense 76
adenomatous polyposis coli 91, 93
adoption 133
Adorno, T.W. 199
adverse drug reactions 212, 232
advisory groups, Sri Lanka 31
Agar, Nicholas 44
All India Institute of Medical
   Sciences 46
amino acid disorders 53
amniocentesis 21-22, 31, 34, 109,
   112, 116, 126, 171, 225
– anxiety 119
– attitudes 118
– disability rights movement in
   Japan 122
– knowledge of 118
– preparation for 112
– risks 34
ancestor worship 132-133

– *senzo sûhai* 127
– family grave 132
– Japan 127
– tatari (punishment) 132
anencephaly 111
antenatal testing 47
anthropological fieldwork 65
anti-sex selection policies
   (China) 226
anxiety 23
– during pregnancy 129
– parental 37
– prenatal genetic testing 129
– testing 30
– 'anxious well' 30
Aryuvedic medicine 48
Asian identity 24
Asian societies 11
astrological horoscope 39
asymptomatic carrier 15
attitudes 104
– Buddhist 36
– Christian 36
– doctors and medical students 32
– to human life 183
– to legal liberalisation of
   termination 34
– to reproductive genetics in
   Japan 131
attitudes to testing 17, 99
– family 17
– society 17
Australian Investment and Financial
   Services Association 161
Ayurvedic medicine 79

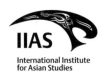

PUBLICATIONS SERIES

International Institute
for Asian Studies

Josine Stremmelaar and Paul van der Velde (eds.)
What about Asia? Revisiting Asian Studies
2006 (ISBN 978 90 5356 959 7)

Monographs

Alex McKay
Their Footprints Remain. Biomedical Beginnings Across the Indo-Tibetan Frontier
Monographs 1
2007 (ISBN 978 90 5356 518 6)

Masae Kato
Women's Rights? The Politics of Eugenic Abortion in Modern Japan
Monographs 2
2009 (ISBN 978 90 5356 793 7)

Jeroen de Kloet
China with a Cut. Globalisation, Urban Youth and Popular Music
Monographs 3
2010 (ISBN 978 90 8964 162 5)

Edited Volumes

Gijsbert Oonk (ed.)
Global Indian Diasporas. Exploring Trajectories of Migration and Theory
Edited Volumes 1
2007 (ISBN 978 90 5356 035 8)

Wen-Shan Yang and Melody Lu (eds.)
Asian Cross-border Marriage Migration. Demographic Patterns and Social Issues
Edited Volumes 2
2010 (ISBN 978 90 8964 054 3)